The We

Spa at Home

The Wellness Center's
Spa at Home

•

Kalia Doner and
Margaret Doner, L. M. T.

with Dale Grust, Director,
The Wellness Center

B

BERKLEY BOOKS / NEW YORK

Acknowledgments

◆

Our heartfelt thanks to Jennifer Lata and Judy Palais for their enthusiasm and guidance, and to our agent, Regula Noetzli, for her ongoing support and dedication.

We'd also like to express our deep appreciation to Dale Montelione Grust, the founder and director of The Wellness Center in Hyde Park, New York, and the Center for Therapeutic Massage in New Paltz, New York; to Maureen DiCorcia, licensed esthetician and certified spa therapist and the director of spa services at The Wellness Center and at the Centre for Well-Being at the Beekman Arms in Rheinbeck, New York; and to Dawn Montelione Scribner, registered dietitian, who was so helpful with the spa cuisine chapter.

KALIA DONER AND
MARGARET DONER, L.M.T.

I'd like to take this opportunity to thank those who have taught, supported, and worked with me over the years and to whom The Wellness Center owes so much:

My mother, who gave me the freedom to follow my heart, the power to know I could succeed, and the support I needed when the road was rocky;

My husband, Jamie, that rare husband who is supportive

but still able to give me the freedom to pursue my career without conflict;

My son, Ryan, who through his early years generously shared me with my career;

Doris Erichson, who gave me the inspiration in 1979 to attend massage school;

Dr. Jay Victor Scherer's Academy of Massage and Natural Healing, where my education was both academic and spiritual;

My sister, Dawn Montelione Scribner, R.D., C.D.N., for her friendship and her substantial contributions to the chapter on nutrition;

Maureen DiCorcia, director of spa services at The Wellness Center, for her hard work on this book;

The massage therapists at The Wellness Center, who bring so much to the book, to the Center, and to my life: Larry Andreassen, Winfield Crans, Margaret Doner, Kerri Fodor, Christian Hanckel, Jennifer Hunderfund, Robin Kozlowski, Maryellen Martinson, Christine Plimley, George Sprauge, and Dawn Ward;

The support staff, past and present, at the Center: Gail Denning, June Wilber, Michaela Strawinski, Jean Murphy, Rebecca Low, and Ann Marie Rivera, who have contributed so much to building and to running the Center—I couldn't have done it without them;

And my loyal clientele, who teach us every day the importance of the will and spirit in the healing process.

DALE MONTELIONE GRUST,
FOUNDER AND DIRECTOR OF THE WELLNESS CENTER
HYDE PARK, NEW YORK

Contents

◆

One

Develop Your Own E.S.P.: Extraordinary Spa Programs for Health and Beauty

As you enter a spa facility, you breathe in the subtle scent of flowers; soft lighting eases you into a dreamy reverie; a serene melody floats by, barely catching your attention. Here, there are no phones, no pressures. You're in an oasis of soothing pleasures. Nearby there's an inviting tub filled with skin-softening emollients. A selection of sensuous skin creams is at your fingertips. Refreshing exotic fruit drinks are available to tease your taste buds. You smile. At last, your mind, your body and your spirit will relax and repair, releasing the harsh stresses that buffet you daily.

Welcome to your spa experience—the perfect remedy for the wear and tear of a sixty-hour workweek; a fight with your fiancé; the endless demands of your two wonderful—but oh so energetic—kids; or that phone call with your mom!

Sound wickedly decadent? Well, it is a bit. But hundreds of thousands of women every year are discovering that this restorative therapy isn't simply an indulgence anymore. Research has shown that chronic stress has serious health repercussions on the immune and cardiovascular systems; holistic healers have long advocated the use of herbal therapies, massage, nutritional discipline and other spa treatments to restore balance in mind and body. And the increasingly sophisticated spa therapies available at the many centers across the country are designed to provide these important physical and spiritual benefits.

Unfortunately, it's often difficult to escape for an afternoon, or longer, to visit a spa facility. But that doesn't mean you have to deny yourself professional-style treatments. The Wellness Center's *Spa at Home* lets you recreate the spa experience. Without leaving the house, you'll be able to evoke the wonderful qualities of the finest spas with music and lighting and scents; you'll concoct the most fabulous facials and body wraps; and you'll delight your palate with delicious spa cuisine, all on your schedule and to suit your whim—and your budget. And you can design your own spa session to create a sensual interlude with your partner, to have fun with your friends, or as a retreat for you alone.

So join us on a journey through your five common senses and their uncommon powers to make you feel and look wonderful. By sampling the spa treatments in this book, you'll cultivate your TASTE with delicious, healthful spa menus that help balance your physical and mental energy.

You'll stimulate your TOUCH, through giving and receiving muscle-soothing massages that help you relax and tune in to your unexpressed feelings.

You'll sharpen your HEARING with guided meditations

that provide an introduction to the ancient art of creating tranquillity in body and spirit.

You'll sweeten your SMELL using sensuous aromatic therapy that practitioners say heals and guides.

You'll focus your SIGHT by increasing your appreciation of the beauty of the human form, a key to increasing your comfort with how you look and feel.

The *Spa at Home* helps you integrate these health-giving spa treatments into your daily and weekly schedule, by offering:

- Facial therapies for every skin type and any schedule—from the five-minute energizing facial to the hour-long restorative treatment
- Quick tricks to repair damaged hair and beautify feet, elbows, hands, nails and eyes
- Soothing soaks to help you ease sore muscles and rest a weary spirit
- Body wraps to cleanse, detoxify, and moisturize you from head to toe
- Basic instructions in partnered and self-massage for every part of your body
- Guided meditations designed to provide you with the tools to create inner tranquillity
- A short course in stretching, and aerobic and muscle-toning exercises
- Delicious spa recipes and menus to help you integrate the health-giving benefits of spa cuisine into your everyday meals

You can enjoy these routines using many of the pre-made formulations available at body shops, but the recipes we provide let you tailor your treatments so they are pure, all natural, and suited to your skin type. In addition, they are a fraction of the cost of commercial products.

So tell the kids to play outside and take the phone off the hook, because you're about to enter the world of personal pleasure and good health.

Two

Face Facts:
The Complete Guide
to At-Home Facials

Facials are the centerpiece of any spa experience. As you lie back in the dimly lit private treatment room, your cares melt away. The healing touch of the person giving you the facial, combined with seemingly magical elixirs, clarifies, revitalizes, and smoothes your skin, restoring a youthful glow. There are few moments as truly relaxing as when your facial is complete and you are left alone to slowly reenter the world.

Why is it so wonderful to have your complexion cleansed, steamed, toned, and moisturized? At The Wellness Center we believe the skin is one of the most important mediums for healing: Your complexion is a mirror of your entire being's physical and spiritual health. Unfortunately, too often the complexion reflects the irritating chemicals, environmental pollutants, fatty foods, and gnawing stress that assault it daily. And the result? Premature wrinkles, clogged pores, irregular skin tone, blotchiness, and/or dry patches.

Luckily, it's never too late to reverse some of the most visible signs. Facials—along with the other at-home spa treatments—can make a dramatic difference in both the appearance and the health of your complexion. Aerobic exercise helps cleanse the skin of surface pollutants and toxins; deep relaxation, meditation, and massage improve cardiovascular health and increase spiritual contentment—which makes you glow; the spa diet eliminates excess fat and calories—and that, too, improves the health of the skin. In addition, the facial treatments in this chapter—*cleansers, compresses, steams, exfoliating scrubs, massage with masks, toners, moisturizers*, and *hydrating moisturizers*—provide targeted care and repair. By spending a few extra minutes a day treating your skin with the respect it deserves, you can take years off your face and increase your self-confidence.

How to Determine Your Skin Type

Before you begin any facial treatment, it's important to determine your skin type. It will guide your choice of cleansers, compresses, steams, scrubs, masks, toners, and moisturizers. The simple three-step plan below will help you identify yours.

Step One: Wash face with a splash of warm water and alcohol-free, soap-free cleanser. See pages 25–28 for suggested formulas.

Step Two: Pull hair back off face. Leave skin free of makeup or creams for a couple of hours.

Step Three: In a well-lit room, swipe the skin with a tissue, particularly around the nose, the brow and chin. Is the tissue clear? You have dry skin. Lightly marked with oil? Your skin is normal. Definitely stained? Your skin is oily.

To refine the evaluation, examine your skin in a well-lit mirror. Do you have blemishes on the nose, cheeks, around the mouth or forehead? Are there dry patches? Identify what areas may be oily or dry. Many people have combination skin, with blemishes and oily and dry patches. If that describes your skin, you'll want to treat each area separately or use products that are made especially for sensitive skin, since combination skin is typically sensitive. So let's get started. It's time to select the facial treatments that are designed specifically for your complexion.

7-Step Facial Basics

·

for each skin type

Skin Care Techniques

When you visit The Wellness Center, or another facility, for a facial, you will experience a series of carefully designed treatments that work together to cleanse and refresh your complexion. Below, we have outlined the seven steps that are used by professional aestheticians: cleansing, compressing, steaming, exfoliating, applying masks, toning, and moisturizing. No matter what the goals are for your skin, these guidelines will give you the basic information you need to treat your skin like a professional.

#1 Cleansing: Washing the face is something we often do without thinking of the consequences. Soap, water and a washcloth are standard fare, but they damage the skin—drying, irritating, and prematurely aging the face. No one should use soap—even the oiliest skin needs to be treated delicately.

How to wash your face
   The basic routine for all skin types is as follows:

+ Wash hands well.
+ Remove eye makeup using cotton balls moistened with gentle cream remover. Avoid alcohol-based products around eyes; the skin there lacks oil and is easily dehydrated.
+ Run warm water on a washcloth. Wring out. Cover face with cloth and allow warmth to loosen dirt and open pores. Repeat. Be very gentle. Don't rub the face with the cloth, skin tissue is delicate and easily damaged.

- Apply cleanser.

  For normal skin, use alcohol-free, non-oily cleansers or a gentle oatmeal cleanser.

  For dry skin, use rich cleansers made from plant-based oils, free of alcohol.

  For oily skin, use oil-free cleansers. Aloe vera gel is soothing, astringent, and purifying.

  For blemished skin, avoid anything that is creamy or abrasive.

  For sensitive or combination skin, use mild perfume-, alcohol-, abrasive-, and color-free milky cleansers.
- Use fingers to gently rub cleansers in a circular motion over skin.
- Rinse well by splashing face with lukewarm water for at least 30 seconds.
- Pat dry with a clean towel, used for your face only.

#2 Compressing: Recommended for daily use by all skin types.

How to make a compress

- Saturate a clean washcloth in water or use the compress recipes on pages 28–30 that are made with herbal teas and essential oils.
- *For normal skin,* cool to lukewarm.
- *For dry skin,* warm.
- *For oily skin,* lukewarm.
- *For blemished, sensitive, or combination skin,* lukewarm water first application, then follow with cool.
- Press the water-saturated cloth over your face so

that the skin is flooded with water and surface dirt is loosened. Hold against skin for the count of five. Rinse cloth and resoak. Apply to face again. Repeat five times.

- When done, gently pat face dry with clean towel.

For herbal and aromatherapy compress recipes see pages 28–30.

#3 Steaming: Recommended for most skin types (acne-prone skin should skip this step), steaming is a deep cleaning technique used to loosen clogs in pores and stimulate blood flow to the skin, which increases nutrients in the area. The frequency, temperature, and length of time you steam are determined by skin type.

To steam clean your face:

- Heat water until just before it breaks into a boil. Pour into basin or large bowl.
- You may add herbs or essential oils to increase the effectiveness of the steam—see recommended recipes on pages 30–31.
- Lean over the basin. Drape towel over your head so that the steam from the basin is concentrated on your face.
- *Normal and oily skin* can take regular steaming, but be careful not to scald skin. Steaming twice a week for up to 10 minutes each time is recommended. See pages 30–31 for more detail.
- *Blemished and sensitive skin*—keep your face at least 12 inches from the steam and limit exposure to three to five minutes. If it helps blemishes and doesn't irritate the skin, you may repeat twice a week.

- *Dry skin* should steam for only a couple minutes. Keep face far enough from steam that the moisture accumulates on the skin but no heat is felt.

#4 *Exfoliating Scrubs:* Recommended, at least occasionally, for all skin types except hypersensitive and acne-prone skin.

Exfoliation is the removal of dead and dry skin. You can do this through the use of a scrub, such as the oatmeal yogurt scrub on page 33 or through the use of natural chemical peelers such as alpha hydroxy acid or papaya enzyme (a milder treatment).

For recipes for scrubs for each skin type see pages 32–35.

#5 *Detoxifying and Moisturizing Masks:* Masks are recommended for all skin types. They should be used at least once a week for 10–20 minutes.

For recipes for your particular skin type, see pages 35–43.

#6 *Toning:* Recommended for all skin types except dry.

Toning is an effective way to remove all residue from cleansing and to restore the Ph balance of the skin. Pure aloe vera gel or juice or diluted cider vinegar are the best universal toners. *(See pages 43–45 for more recipes.)* Apply toner with a damp cotton ball.

#7 *Moisturizing:* Recommended for most skin types —oily and blemished skin need specialized formulations. (Acne-prone skin may need to avoid moisturizing, since it may provoke breakouts.)

Designed to hold in moisture and/or provide oil to skin, moisturizers are essential for fighting off premature wrinkles and dull, lifeless-looking skin. They should be used at least once a day, particularly around eyes and upper lip.

Normal Skin

Normal skin is neither too oily nor too dry. Your goal is to keep it well hydrated and to avoid damage from harsh cleansers, pollutants, and the sun.

Care Routine

- *Cleanse* with alcohol-free, non-soapy cleansers. The *oatmeal cleanser* on page 25 is ideal for daily use.
- *Compress* every day with a warm or cool cloth. You may want to add to the basin of water 5 drops of essential oils, such as chamomile or ylang-ylang; or 2 cups strong chamomile or peppermint tea.
- *Steam* twice a week with a mild herbal steam, such as chamomile, for no more than five minutes. Be careful not to scald skin. Use essential oils and teas on pages 30–31 to increase the effectiveness of the steams.
- *Scrubs* and exfoliants can be used daily if they're not too drying or abrasive. Try the *oatbran egg yolk scrub* on page 32. And be careful not to rub hard! You may also choose an alpha-hydroxy acid product to diminish fine lines. If redness or dry patches appear, discontinue for a few days and then select a milder concentration.

- *Masks* can be used weekly to keep skin glowing and well nourished. Clay- or seaweed-based masks will rid the skin of toxins, but they can be drying (which is particularly hard on aging skin), so you might alternate them with moisturizing masks such as the *avocado mask* on page 36.
- *Toners* should be used after every wash to remove cleanser residue and reestablish Ph balance. The *cucumber toner* on page 44 is the perfect balancer. Other possibilities: a splash of floral water, or the *witch hazel lemon-mint toner* on page 44.
- *Moisturizers* are essential for all skin types; they help the skin screen out external pollutants and keep the skin hydrated, which helps prevent wrinkles. The trick is finding a moisturizer that doesn't feel greasy or clog pores. For the daytime, use a light alcohol-free lotion and for nighttime try the *vitamin E treatment* on page 45. As you age, you may want to increase the amount of moisturizer you use—particularly concentrating specially formulated eye creams on the skin around the eyes and upper lip.

Dry Skin

Dry skin suffers from lack of moisture and/or lack of oil. Often there are blemishes around the dry patches. Treating dry skin calls for a delicate balance between providing enough moisture and oil and not using so many emollients that you'll end up blocking the pores.

Care Routine

- *Cleansing* needs to be done only once a day—in the morning you can simply splash your face with warm water and

Aromatherapy

Essential oils used in aromatherapy are extracted essences of plants that contain hormones, vitamins, antibiotics and antiseptics. They impact the mind, body and spirit through their aroma and their chemical properties. Used for cosmetic purposes, they can help balance and soothe your skin. The essential oils that we recommend throughout the various sections of this book for use in compresses, steaming, cleansing, moisturizers, and masks are generally safe, although pregnant women should always be cautious and check with their doctor and an aromatherapy specialist before using. They should always avoid juniper, basil and peppermint oils.

In this book we recommend the following:

◆ chamomile	◆ orange	◆ ylang-ylang	◆ basil
◆ geranium	◆ lavender	◆ peppermint	◆ bergamot
◆ juniper	◆ eucalyptus	◆ carrot	
◆ avocado	◆ cabbage	◆ rose	

Never use any essential oil straight from the bottle. Add essential oils to a carrier such as aloe vera gel or vegetable oil before using (2–3 drops per teaspoon or 15–20 drops to ¼ cup). It is not recommended that you use any essential oil for more than two or three weeks.

Beware of those that are potentially toxic. Rue, thuja, mugwort, sage, hyssop, anise and fennel are perhaps the most dangerous. The International Federation of Aromatherapists has a list of more than 35 oils that it considers unwise to use. To obtain a copy write: 4 Eastmearn Rd., Dulwich, London, SE21 8HA England.

pat dry. Then apply moisturizer. In the evening, remove makeup with a gentle, water-based, alcohol-free product. The oatmeal milk cleanser on page 27 is nonirritating and moisturizing. Rinse with warm water and pat dry.

- *Compress* dry skin twice a day with a cloth soaked in warm water. Once a day add 5–10 drops of carrot or avocado essential oil to the basin of water.

- *Steaming* is hard on dry skin even though it needs the moisture. Limit it to once a month. Apply moisturizer to skin before steaming and use for 2–3 minutes, keeping your face about 12 inches from the source of the steam.

- *Exfoliation* can be important if dry skin is dull. The trick is to remove that surface layer of dead cells without damaging the dry skin. The best approach is to use the *oatbran egg yolk scrub* on page 32 no more than once a month.

- *Masks* can be wonderfully nurturing—stick with those that moisturize, such as the *honey almond oil mask* on page 38. You can use a mask once a week, if your skin responds positively.

- *Toners* can be too harsh for dry skin, so use a very dilute solution of cider vinegar and water to restore acid balance, and then apply moisturizer.

- *Moisturize* with a creamy, alcohol-free product around eyes and upper lip. Vitamin E (page 45) is useful at night for extra dry areas. You can purchase a cream that is a humectant (water retaining) for the rest of your face. And always drink eight glasses of water a day.

Oily Skin

Oily skin may be more wrinkle resistant that other types, but it's also blemish prone and if overtreated may develop dry patches. The goal is to keep pores from clogging and to restore balance.

Care Routine

- *Cleansing* should not be done more than twice a day since it can cause excess oil production and dry patches. If your skin feels oily during the day, blot it gently with cotton pads. Or if you're really desperate: Refresh with a spray of 1 part witch hazel and 3 parts water and then blot face. (Keep your eyes closed!) Morning and night cleanse with pure aloe vera gel or the *lemon honey aloe vera wash* on page 27. When done, splash face with cool water. Pat dry.
- *Compresses* should be warm to cool. Make them from either green or chamomile tea or 5–10 drops of geranium, lavender, or cabbage essential oils (see pages 28–30).
- *Steaming* is important twice a week since it rids the pores of oil buildup. Recommended are the *lemon balm, sage,* and *chamomile herbal tea steams* on pages 30–31. But you want to make sure you rebalance the skin's Ph by using a toner.
- *Exfoliation* is helpful in controlling oily skin. To open up clogged pores use either an alpha-hydroxy acid product or the *oatbran egg yolk scrub* on page 32.
- *Masks* made with *clay, cucumber, egg white,* and *seaweed,* pages 35–43, help eliminate excess oil.
- *Toners* are important to rebalance the skin—once your face is well cleaned and the oil has been removed from the surface area. Especially good is the *witch hazel lemon-mint toner* on page 44 and the *cucumber toner* on page 44. You may also buy a commercially made, alcohol-free product.
- *Moisturizers* should be used around the eyes even if you

have oily skin. Vitamin E is always simple and effective. As for the rest of your face, at night use an oil-free lotion or aloe vera gel.

Blemished Skin

Blemishes can happen to anyone at any age. They may be a result of food allergies, sensitivities to external irritants, excess oil production, plugged oil ducts, hormonal fluctuations, or bacteria. But whatever the cause, they require special care. Those of you with sensitive skin that blemishes easily should follow the recommendations in this section. Combination skin? Use treatments appropriate to skin conditions in various areas of your face.

Care Routine

- *Cleansing* should be done with a fresh washcloth twice a day. Beware of scrubbing or overcleaning and choose a cleanser that doesn't leave a potentially irritating residue. Cream cleansers are not a good idea—experiment with gentle foaming gels or rely on pure aloe vera gel—guaranteed to help heal irritated skin.

  If you want to use an aromatherapy-based cleanser, the essential oils recommended for acne include bergamot, eucalyptus, juniper (not for pregnant women), and lavender. They may be mixed with aloe vera to form a cleansing lotion or you can use the *essential chamomile oil–aloe vera gel* method described on page 25.

- *Compresses* should be done first with a lukewarm cloth soaked in a basin of water infused with *lemon balm* or *chamomile tea* or *eucalyptus* or *lavender essential oil* (see pages 28–30). You may also want to use a floral water—available at all body and bath shops. It's gentler than essential oils and still effective. *Make sure not to get these essential oil compresses in your eyes.* Finish compress with cool water.

- *Steam* for 3–5 minutes a couple times a week to cleanse pores and moisturize your face. Remember to keep your face about 12 inches from the source of the steam. You may want to infuse the water with aromatics such as cabbage and juniper (not for pregnant women) essential oils or herbal teas such as *chamomile* or *lemon balm* (see pages 30–31). Or better yet—to warm the face and unclog the pores, drink 8 glasses of water a day and make sure you get regular, vigorous aerobic exercise.

- *Exfoliation* can help clear up pimples but you should never scrub or irritate inflamed skin. Instead, try the skin-peeling powers of alpha-hydroxy acid or papaya enzyme. Make sure you don't use too strong a solution.

- *Masks* can be extremely helpful—particularly clay masks that help dry up pimples. Use as often as you can without drying skin. A *banana chamomile mask* (page 42) can soothe, and a coating of plain honey can help blemishes go away more quickly.

- *Toner* for blemished skin should calm the irritation—the *aloe vera chamomile splash* on page 45 is particularly effective.

- *Moisturizers* may only aggravate the blemishes—look for moisturizers designed especially for blemished skin. If you have dry skin in some areas, try using aloe vera gel all by itself to bring moisture to the skin or use vitamin E—sparingly. It helps healing as well as being a super moisturizer.

Facial Recipes

◆

for cleansers, compresses, steams,
exfoliating scrubs, masks, toners,
and moisturizers

Cleansers

Cleansers are designed to remove surface dirt without drying or irritating the skin. For information about what kind of cleanser to use and how to apply it, see How to Wash Your Face on pages 11–12.

Aloe vera gel is a universal cleanser for dry, oily, normal, and blemished skin. Used straight or with a few drops of chamomile essential oil (in 2 tablespoons of aloe vera), it will remove surface dirt, soothe the skin, prevent loss of moisture, and absorb excess oil.

CLEANSERS FOR NORMAL SKIN

Use one of the following daily cleansers:

Oatmeal Cleanser

*

½ cup oatmeal
¾ cup hot water
1 tablespoon olive oil

Combine ingredients in blender until smooth and let sit until oatmeal has absorbed much of the water. It will remain a thick liquid. Use like soap. Keep leftovers in the refrigerator.

Remember: For all spa treatments made from perishable ingredients:
*   Store leftovers in the refrigerator.*

♦ Never use anything that you suspect has lost its freshness.

Yogurt and Honey Cleanser

♦

4 ounces plain whole milk yogurt
2 tablespoons honey
1 tablespoon canola oil

Combine ingredients in blender. Coat face with mixture and then using fingers massage face well. Rinse in cool to warm water. Repeat. (This combination makes a lovely body wash in the shower as well—pour on washcloth and massage into thighs, arms, and torso. Rinse.) Can be stored in the refrigerator for 2–3 days.

CLEANSERS FOR DRY SKIN

Cocoa Butter Cream Cleanser

♦

1 tablespoon cocoa butter
½ teaspoon coconut oil (you may use an odorless oil as well; avoid olive, walnut, almond)
1 teaspoon cornmeal or ground raw oatmeal

Mix ingredients together in the palm of your hand or a small bowl and apply to damp face. Allow to sit for a minute or so. Splash face repeatedly with warm water. Wipe off with damp cotton balls. Pat dry with towel.

Oatmeal Milk Cleanser

•

½ cup ground raw oatmeal
¼ cup hot water
¼ cup half-and-half (or whole milk)

Combine ingredients in a blender until creamy. Smooth over face and use fingertips to massage skin gently. Rinse with warm water. Reapply. Let sit for 1 minute. Rinse with cool water several times. Pat dry with towel.

CLEANSERS FOR OILY SKIN

Lemon, Honey, Aloe Vera Wash

•

2 tablespoons pure aloe vera gel
1 teaspoon fresh lemon juice
1 teaspoon honey

Combine ingredients well and apply to face moistened with warm to hot water. Use fingertips or a soft cosmetic sponge to massage the face. Keep lemon juice out of eyes. Rinse well with warm water.

Tomato Cucumber Cleanser

•

1 ripe tomato (optional)
½ medium cucumber
1 teaspoon oil

Peel the cucumber and remove the seeds. Blend and then strain through tea strainer. Save juice. Chop ripe tomato into very small bits. Strain. Combine with cucumber juice and oil.

Apply to damp face. Place warm washcloth over face and gently wipe off the cleanser. Repeat. Rinse.

CLEANSERS FOR BLEMISHED SKIN

Use gentle, mildly antiseptic cleansers.

Peppermint Yogurt Bath

♦

2 tablespoons skim milk yogurt
5 drops peppermint essential oil (not for pregnant women)

Add essential oil to yogurt and mix well. Apply to face using the palm and extended fingers of both hands. Don't rub, glide gently. Allow cleanser to sit on face for 1 minute. Splash face with warm water. Pat dry with clean towel.

Aloe Vera Aromatherapy Cleanser

♦

¼ cup aloe vera gel
3–4 drops lavender oil with or without bergamot
     (2 drops of each) or
3 drops of eucalyptus essential oil (by itself)

Mix ingredients together well and rub gently over damp face. Rinse with warm water.

Compresses

Compresses are designed to loosen surface dirt and gently unclog pores. For basic guidelines see How to Make a Compress, on page 12. The recipes given below are for compresses made with herbal teas or essential oils.

Beyond the Basics

Essential oil compress: Mix 5–10 drops of essential oil with 1 teaspoon of vinegar. This helps the oil mix more evenly in the water and avoids the problem of exposure to full-strength essential oils.

Add the oil and vinegar to the quart of warm water in which you are going to soak the washcloth.

Herbal tea compress: Fill the sink with about 1 quart of water: lukewarm water for inflamed or blemished skin; warm for dry skin; lukewarm for oily skin; and lukewarm to cool for normal skin. Pour in 2 cups of herbal tea steeped for 10–20 minutes and strained. You can make the tea using a ¼ cup of fresh or a tablespoon of dried herbs.

Compresses for Normal Skin

Use ylang-ylang, geranium, or lavender essential oils, or peppermint (not for pregnant women), fennel, or chamomile tea.

Compresses for Dry Skin

Use parsley and chamomile tea with 2 tablespoons of honey. Using aromatherapy essential oils? Try peppermint (not for pregnant women), rose, or carrot.

Compresses for Oily Skin

Use sage, chamomile, or lemon balm tea. Essential oils that are good for oily skin include geranium, ylang-ylang, lavender, and basil (not for pregnant women).

Compresses for Blemished and Sensitive Skin

Use a tea made from chamomile, lemon balm, valerian, or lime flowers. Essential oils that can be used include eucalyptus, juniper (not for pregnant women), and lavender; chamomile and floral waters are good for highly sensitive skin.

Steams

Steaming is good for all skin types—depending on how close you are to the steam and the length of time you spend. For basic guidelines for each skin type, see page 13.

> Tip: *Always be careful not to scald the skin. And remember to put a thin layer of rich cream around eyes and on lips before steaming.*

Steaming for Normal Skin

Normal skin can take the full force of the steam, but be careful not to overdo it. If the steam burns the inside of your nose when you inhale, you're way too close to the source—move back several inches.

Herbal steams: 1 cup fresh or 3 tablespoons dried chamomile, fennel, or rosemary, tied in cheesecloth or an old stocking and steeped in 1 gallon boiling water.

Essential oil–based steams: Use between 5 and 15 drops of lavender, ylang-ylang, carrot, lemon (not for sensitive or allergic skin), or geranium.

Steaming for Dry Skin

Dry skin should steam for no more than 2–3 minutes and the face should be several inches from the source of the steam so that the moisture accumulates on the skin but no heat is felt.

Herbal steams: 1 cup fresh or 3 tablespoons dried parsley or chamomile.

Essential oil–based steams: Use 5–15 drops of peppermint (not for use during pregnancy), carrot, or chamomile.

Steaming for Blemished Skin

Blemished and sensitive skin should steam for 3–5 minutes and the face should be 12 inches from the source of the steam.

Herbal steams: Use 1 cup fresh or 3 tablespoons dried chamomile or lemon balm per gallon of water.

Essential oil–based steams: Use 5–15 drops of lavender, eucalyptus, or bergamot per gallon of water.

Steaming for Oily Skin

Oily skin may need deep cleansing, but too much heat can overstimulate oil glands. Keep face about 16 inches from surface of water so it's a gentle, warm mist. Don't let skin become red or hot to the touch.

Herbal steams: 1 cup fresh or 3 tablespoons of dried sage, chamomile, lemon balm, or lime flowers per gallon of water.

Essential oil–based steams: Use between 5 and 15 drops of lavender, geranium, basil (not for use during pregnancy), ylang-ylang, or lemon (not for sensitive or allergic skin).

Scrubs and Exfoliation

Scrubs and exfoliation clear off dead and dry skin cells and bring luster and tone to your complexion. Some are designed for use once a week or even less frequently. But others are mild enough to use daily. If you have sensitive skin that reacts unpredictably, turns red or develops rashes, or is acne-prone, skip the scrubs.

> *Normal, dry, and oily skin can all use a scrub made from ground oatmeal, hot water, and olive oil. Mix together a small palmful of finely ground oatmeal, 1–2 tablespoons of hot water and a few drops of oil. Splash face with water and then massage with oat mixture. Let sit on skin for 1 minute. Rinse with cool water. Then dab skin with cider vinegar and water solution (1 part vinegar to 4 parts water).*

GENTLE SCRUBS FOR NORMAL SKIN
Use a mild scrub to cleanse and moisturize.

Oatbran Egg Yolk Scrub
◆

1 egg yolk* (Save the egg white for a mask.)
½ cup oatbran, precooked and cooled
2 teaspoons canola oil (or almond or avocado)

Cook oatbran and allow to cool. Stir in raw egg yolk and oil. Dip your fingers in the mixture and spread on your damp face. Massage gently with fingertips, then rinse well with luke-warm water.

*You may substitute 3 tablespoons honey or use oatmeal and oil alone.

Almond Honey Cream Scrub

•

1–2 tablespoons ground almonds
1 tablespoon honey
2 tablespoons whole milk plain yogurt

Grind nuts in blender or food processor. Add to mixture of honey and yogurt. Spread over damp face and massage with fingertips. Rinse thoroughly with warm water. Pat dry with towel.

CREAMY SCRUBS FOR DRY SKIN

Use a creamy scrub once a week to cleanse and moisturize.

Oatmeal Yogurt Scrub

•

2 tablespoons oil (canola, olive, almond, or avocado)
3 tablespoons oatmeal
½ teaspoon fresh lemon juice
1 tablespoon whole milk yogurt

Grind oatmeal in a blender until in small bits, but still coarse. Mix all ingredients together until smooth and well blended. Apply to damp face. Let sit for 1 minute. Massage with fingertips. Rinse off with lukewarm water. You can keep any leftover scrub in the refrigerator for 2–3 days.

Sugar Scrub

◆

...poons granulated sugar
1 tablespoon avocado, almond, or canola oil
1 teaspoon cream

Combine ingredients in a small bowl. Spread on damp face and massage gently with fingertips. Rinse off with lukewarm water. Pat dry.

SCRUBS FOR OILY SKIN

Use an oil-free scrub to cleanse every other day.

Aloe Vera Oatmeal Scrub

◆

¼ cup ground oatmeal
¼ cup water
2 tablespoons aloe vera gel

Grind raw oatmeal in a blender until in small pieces, but still coarse. Pour water over oatmeal and stir. Allow to sit until water is somewhat absorbed. Add aloe vera gel; stir well. Spread on damp face with fingertips and massage all over with a gently circular motion. Rinse off with warm water and repeat. Rinse and pat dry.

Banana Cornmeal Scrub

◆

½ ripe banana
2–3 tablespoons cornmeal

Mash the banana and stir in the cornmeal. Spread the mixture over your face and massage into skin with your fin-

gertips. Rinse with warm water. Repeat if desired. Rinse and
pat dry.

SCRUBS FOR BLEMISHED SKIN

Abrasive scrubs—even oatmeal—can be too rough on
blemished skin. Better to opt for an exfoliating product with
alpha-hydroxy acid or papaya enzymes.

Masks

Masks are a special part of the spa treatment process—there
is something so soothing about relaxing while they do their
deep cleaning and moisturizing. You should give yourself an
appropriate mask once a week, no matter what skin type you
have.

For all of these applications, prepare the treatment mixture and then stretch out. You'll want to apply them while
you're reclining, so they don't run. We suggest that you use
the opportunity to enjoy a complimentary spa treatment such
as a foot soak, a meditation, or perhaps to have your spa
partner give you a hand or foot massage.

Tip: Be careful not to get any of these masks in your
eyes. *We recommend that you make a strong cup of
chamomile tea and soak four to six cotton balls in the
liquid. Squeeze them out so they're still wet, but not dripping, and place them in the refrigerator for a couple of
minutes until chilled. Place one over each eye and sit back
and relax while the masks work their magic. Replace with
cool cotton balls as you like.*

Oatmeal again takes the prize as the best basic ingredient—every skin type can benefit from an oatmeal-based mask.

- For normal skin, combine ¼ cup *cooked* oatmeal, 1 egg, and 1 tablespoon of oil.
- For oily skin, to cooked oatmeal add 1 egg white blended with a dash of grapefruit or lemon juice or 2 drops of lavender or ylang-ylang essential oil.
- For dry skin, add to the cooked oatmeal 2 tablespoons honey, 2 drops wheat germ oil (or peppermint—*not for pregnant women*—or carrot essential oil) mixed with 1 tablespoon of canola oil. Spread on your face and let set for 10 minutes. Rinse off with cool water. Pat dry.

MASKS FOR NORMAL SKIN

Use a mask every week to cleanse and hydrate your complexion.

Avocado Mask

◆

½ ripe avocado
1–2 teaspoons fresh lemon juice

Cream the avocado and mix in the lemon juice. Spread a thin layer over clean skin. Allow to dry for 10–15 minutes. Wash off with lukewarm water.

*Tip: To apply a liquid mask, use a basting brush or clean
paintbrush about 1½–2 inches wide.*

Jell-O Surprise

◆

*1 tablespoon plain gelatin
2 ounces distilled or spring water
2 ounces coconut milk or cream of coconut**

Cook gelatin and liquids over low heat until gelatin is well
dissolved. Cool—in the refrigerator it goes faster—until it
starts congealing. In a reclining position, spread over face and
allow to sit for 15 minutes. Peel off and rinse face with lukewarm water.

*You may substitute organic apple juice, whole milk, or 2 ounces of chamomile
tea.

Fruit Moisturizing Mask

◆

*½ banana
1 ripe pear or ¼ cup pear juice
1 tablespoon coconut, avocado or almond oil
    (if not available use canola oil)
3 tablespoons honey*

Puree banana and pear or pear juice in blender. Add the
honey and 1 tablespoon oil. Mix well. Spread on face and
allow to sit for 15–20 minutes. Store leftovers in airtight sterile
jar in refrigerator for up to a week.

Tip: If you have food allergies, avoid using masks or any other treatments that contain those foods.

Seaweed Detoxifying Mask

◆

If you can't buy a packaged seaweed mask at your local drugstore, you can make your own.

2 tablespoons kelp powder
¼ cup aloe vera gel
water

Combine the kelp and aloe in a blender or mixing bowl. Add water very slowly until you arrive at a smooth, thick consistency.

Aromatherapy Mask

◆

To the basic oatmeal, fruit, or any ready-made clay mask, add 1 teaspoon of vegetable oil or aloe vera gel blended with 5 drops of avocado, wheat germ, or chamomile essential oil.

MASKS FOR DRY SKIN

Use a mask once a week—or more—to bring moisture and oils to the skin.

Honey Almond Oil Mask

◆

2 tablespoons honey
1 tablespoon almond oil

Mix honey and oil and spread over clean face. Leave on for 20 minutes. Rinse off with lukewarm water.

Olive Oil, Egg and Lemon Mask

◆

1 egg yolk
1 tablespoon olive oil
2–3 drops lemon juice

Whisk vigorously until smooth. Let sit for 5–10 minutes. Apply to clean skin and allow to sit for 10 minutes. Rinse with lukewarm water. **Note:** You can also use this formula for dry hair and scalp.

Mayonnaise Super-rich Mask

◆

3 tablespoons mayonnaise
1 teaspoon vitamin E oil

Combine ingredients and apply to clean face. Leave on for 10 minutes. Wipe off with cotton balls soaked in warm water. Splash face with water and pat dry.

Milk and Cookies Mask

◆

2 tablespoons heavy cream
1 egg
1 teaspoon almond flour or super-fine gravy flour
1 teaspoon honey

Whisk together ingredients until well blended. Using a basting brush or brand-new paintbrush, swab mixture over skin. Allow to dry for 15 minutes. Rinse off with cool water.

Aromatherapy Mask

◆

To the basic oatmeal, fruit, or any ready-made clay mask, add 1 teaspoon olive, avocado, almond, or canola oil blended with 5 drops of peppermint (not for pregnant women) or ylang-ylang essential oil.

MASKS FOR OILY SKIN

Use a mask once or twice a week to reduce oiliness and clear clogged pores.

Yogurt Meringue

◆

¼ cup low-fat plain yogurt
6–8 drops lemon juice
1 egg white

Whip the egg white until it forms stiff peaks. Fold in yogurt and lemon juice. Apply to clean face. Leave on for 10 minutes. Rinse off with warm water.

Egg White, Aloe, Lavender Mask

◆

2 egg whites
2 tablespoons of aloe vera gel
5 drops of lavender essential oil

Beat egg whites until they reach the soft peak stage. Mix lavender oil with aloe vera gel. Fold into the egg whites, turning over whites until the ingredients are smooth and well blended. Reclining, apply to clean face. Allow to sit until egg white dries. Rinse well with lukewarm water.

Lemon Zest Banana Mask

◆

1 ripe banana
2 tablespoons lemon juice
1 teaspoon lemon zest

Blend banana with lemon juice. Grate lemon skin. Add zest to mixture. Spread on face and allow to sit for 15 minutes. Rinse with lukewarm water.

Cucumber Mask

◆

1 small cucumber
1 packet gelatin
2 ounces chamomile tea
2 ounces distilled water

Peel, seed, and puree cucumber. Pour through fine sieve or coffee filter. In a saucepan, add gelatin to cucumber juice along with 2 ounces chamomile tea and 2 ounces distilled water. Stir well and heat on stove to help dissolve gelatin. Cool in refrigerator half an hour or less, until it has begun to congeal. Recline and spread on face with fingers. Allow to dry for at least 15 minutes. Peel off and then wipe face with cotton balls moistened with distilled water. Pat dry.

Aromatherapy Mask

◆

c oatmeal, fruit or any ready-made clay mask, add
ⅎ ιₑₐₛₚoon aloe vera gel blended with 5 drops of lavender,
geranium, ylang-ylang essential oil.

MASKS FOR BLEMISHED SKIN

Use a mask once a week or more to remove toxins and
soothe irritation.

Beta-Carotene Mask

◆

2 tablespoons carrot juice
1/4 cup aloe vera gel

Mix carrot juice with aloe vera gel. Allow to sit at room
temperature for 5 minutes. Apply to face and let sit for 20
minutes. Rinse well with warm water.

Banana Chamomile Soother

◆

1 ripe banana
2 tablespoons strong chamomile tea
4 cotton balls

Mix banana and tea together until smooth paste is formed.
Dip cotton ball in mixture and swab gently over blemishes.
Take 2 fresh cotton balls and dip in mixture. Place over irritated areas. Let sit for 5 minutes. Rinse off with cool water
and use remaining cotton ball to swab away gently any remaining mask.

Tomato Astringent Mask

◆

2 tablespoons tomato paste
4 thin slices fresh tomato
1 tablespoon aloe vera gel

Mix tomato paste and aloe vera gel. Slice tomato. Spread a thin layer of the aloe mixture on skin. Recline comfortably. Place sliced tomatoes over blemished areas. Allow to sit for 10 minutes. Rinse off with lukewarm water.

Aromatherapy Mask

◆

To the basic oatmeal, banana, or any ready-made clay mask, add 1 teaspoon olive, avocado, almond, or canola oil blended with 5 drops of lavender and bergamot essential oil.

Toners

Toners should be used after cleansing to remove any residue, close pores, and restore balance to skin. They are generally used for dry skin only in super-dilute solution and are always alcohol-free.

Cider vinegar diluted with spring water is a good toner for all skin types. Its acidity helps restore the shield that protects the skin from outside contaminants. Mix 2 tablespoons of vinegar in 1 cup of spring water. Apply to face with cotton balls. Avoid eye area.

TONERS FOR NORMAL OR OILY SKIN

You may use one of the following daily toners:

Witch Hazel Lemon-Mint Toner

◆

½ cup springwater
¼ cup witch hazel
1 tablespoon lemon juice
½ cup well-steeped peppermint tea

In a sterile 12-ounce bottle combine ingredients. Keeps refrigerated for 2 days or divide into smaller containers for freezing. Apply with cotton balls moistened.

Cucumber Toner

◆

This is a mildly astringent toner.

1 large cucumber
3 tablespoons witch hazel
2 tablespoons water

Peel and seed the cucumber. Place in blender until pulverized. Strain the liquid through a fine sieve or coffee filter. Add witch hazel and water to the juice you collect. Apply to face using cotton pads. Keeps refrigerated for several days.

TONER FOR BLEMISHED SKIN

Use the following toner daily:

Aloe Vera Chamomile Splash

•

¼ cup aloe vera gel
3 drops of chamomile essential oil
   or 1 tablespoon of very strong chamomile tea

Combine ingredients and apply to face with damp cotton balls.

Moisturizers

Moisturizers are important for all skin types, particularly around the eyes and the upper lip. There are many wonderful products available—made especially for each skin type. We have included a few make-your-own recipes, but by and large your best bet is to spend some time reading the labels at your local drugstore or bath shop until you find one that sounds right for you. If you have oily or blemished skin look for oil-free moisturizers, and all skin types can use humectants—that is, water-attracting lotions. Among nature's most water-attracting substances: pears, most berries, and plums.

Vitamin E oil takes the prize as the best all-round mois-turizer—but it may seem too sticky to use during the day. So we suggest you blend it with your favorite eye cream and overall moisturizer—about 3 drops of vitamin E oil to a tablespoon of cream should do it, but you'll need to experiment to see what the correct proportion is for your particular creams. At night you can daub pure vi-tamin E right on your skin—remember a very little bit goes a long way. If you have oily skin, you probably won't

want to use it all over your face—but you could apply it
to any irritated or dry patches that may appear. Those
with blemished skin can add it to aloe vera gel for a
soothing, healing application.

Moisturizers for Normal Skin

You may not need an all-over moisturizer, but your eyes, cheeks, and neck should have a light alcohol-free moisturizer every day.

Essential oils that can be added to basic unscented creams or carrier lotions available at most bath and beauty shops include chamomile, lavender, and ylang-ylang. Add only a few drops to every 2 ounces so the aroma is subtle. (Excess ylang-ylang can cause nausea.)

Moisturizers for Dry Skin

A moisturizer is essential morning and night, but you want to guard against clogging your pores. You should always look for products that are labeled as humectants—your skin is thirsty.

Essential oils that can be added to basic unscented creams or carrier lotions available at most bath and beauty shops include rose and carrot.

Moisturizers for Oily Skin

Use a moisturizer only around eyes and on any dry patches that may appear. As you age, dehydration may become a problem—in that case use an oil-free moisturizer. Applied at night, aloe vera gel will provide moisture without oil.

Essential oils that can be added to aloe vera gel include

lavender, bergamot, ylang-ylang, and geranium. Add only a few drops to every 2 ounces so the aroma is subtle.

Moisturizers for Blemished Skin

Moisturizer should be oil-free and slightly antiseptic. Use as needed.

Essential oils that can be added to aloe vera or nonirritating lotions available at most bath and beauty shops include lavender, bergamot, rose, and carrot.

Facial Routines

·

for 5-, 30-, and 60-minute
treatments

Facials for Every Need and Every Schedule

When you visit a spa facility, your aesthetician presents you with a menu of facial routines to choose from. Some are designed to provide a quick pick-me-up, others target specific skin problems, and they all offer a soothing session of pampering and relaxation. Now you have the same delightful choices at home.

In this section we outline 5-, 30-, and 60-minute facials and the full array of treatments you can use for each. You can, of course, substitute any of the other appropriate recipes in this chapter—for cleansers, compresses, steams, scrubs, masks, toners and moisturizers—that suit your mood and schedule. We've tried to give you a template to follow so that you'll always be able to find the time to enjoy taking care of your complexion.

Tip: You can use any of these routines for a back or derriere treatment if you have blemishes or your skin is not as smooth as you'd like it to be.

5-Minute Facials

You can't do everything in five minutes, but you can refresh your skin and help clear away the day's stress and grime. Below are the basics for three types of 5-minute facials: energizing, cleansing, and moisturizing. They'll bring a glow to your skin and a smile to your face.

5-Minute Facials to Enliven and Energize

	FOR NORMAL SKIN	FOR DRY SKIN	FOR OILY SKIN	FOR BLEMISHED SKIN
Step One: Cleanser	oatmeal	oatmeal milk	lemon, honey, aloe	peppermint yogurt
Step Two: Compress	peppermint tea	chamomile tea and honey	sage tea	chamomile tea
Step Three: Toner	witch hazel lemon-mint	diluted cider vinegar	witch hazel lemon-mint	aloe chamomile
Step Four: Moisturizer	light eye cream	carrot and rose essential oils in alcohol-free cream; drink 32 ounces of springwater	oil-free cream	2–3 drops of lavender and bergamot essential oils in 3 tablespoons aloe vera gel

5-Minute Facials to Cleanse

	FOR NORMAL SKIN	FOR DRY SKIN	FOR OILY SKIN	FOR BLEMISHED SKIN
Step One: *Cleanser*	oatmeal	oatmeal milk	lemon, honey, aloe	peppermint yogurt
Step Two: *Steam*	rosemary tea	chamomile tea	chamomile tea	lavender and bergamot essential oils
Step Three: *Scrub*	oatbran egg yolk	sugar scrub	aloe oatmeal	exfoliants such as alpha-hydroxy acid or papaya enzyme
Step Four: *Moisturizer*	light eye cream	carrot and rose essential oils in alcohol-free cream	oil-free cream	2–3 drops of lavender and bergamot essential oils in 3 tablespoons aloe vera gel

5-Minute Facials to Moisturize

	FOR NORMAL SKIN	FOR DRY SKIN	FOR OILY SKIN	FOR BLEMISHED SKIN
Step One: *Cleanser*	yogurt aloe	cocoa butter	lemon, honey, aloe	peppermint yogurt
Step Two: *Mask*	avocado	mayonnaise	banana lemon	banana avocado
Step Three: *Toner*	diluted cider vinegar	diluted cider vinegar	diluted cider vinegar	diluted cider vinegar
Step Four: *Moisturizer*	alcohol-free cream	vitamin E oil	oil-free cream	2–3 drops lavender and bergamot essential oils in 3 tablespoons aloe vera gel

The 30-Minute Facial

In half an hour you can provide your skin with a terrifically renewing experience that incorporates many of the treatments that you get in a full treatment.

	FOR NORMAL SKIN	FOR DRY SKIN	FOR OILY SKIN	FOR BLEMISHED SKIN
Step One: Cleanser	yogurt honey	cocoa butter cream	tomato cucumber	peppermint yogurt
Step Two: Compress	chamomile	chamomile	sage tea or ylang-ylang essential oil	chamomille
Step Three: Steam—3 minutes	chamomile	chamomile	chamomile	chamomile
Step Four: Mask—5 minutes	avocado	honey almond	egg white, aloe	tomato astringent
Step Five: Toner	witch hazel lemon-mint	diluted cider vinegar	diluted cider vinegar	aloe chamomile splash or cider vinegar
Step Six: Moisturizer	alcohol-free light cream	vitamin E oil	oil-free cream	lavender essential oil in aloe gel

The 60-Minute Facial

If you can set aside an hour for your facial, you will be able to indulge in all the steps—and you'll find you feel like you've been on holiday.

	FOR NORMAL SKIN	FOR DRY SKIN	FOR OILY SKIN	FOR BLEMISHED SKIN
Step One: *Cleanser*	yogurt honey	oatmeal milk	lemon, honey, aloe vera	peppermint yogurt
Step Two: *Compress*	chamomile tea	chamomile and honey	chamomile	chamomile
Step Three: *Cleanser, again*	yogurt oatmeal	oatmeal milk	lemon, honey, aloe vera	peppermint yogurt
Step Four: *Steam*	ylang-ylang essential oil	carrot essential oil	lavender essential oil	eucalyptus essential oil
Step Five: *Scrub*	oatmeal egg	sugar scrub	aloe oatmeal	do not use
Step Six: *Mask*	avocado	honey almond	mayonnaise and vitamin E	beta-carotene
Step Seven: *Toner*	cucumber	diluted cider vinegar	witch hazel lemon-mint	aloe chamomile
Step Eight: *Moisturize*	a lotion with ylang-ylang essential oil	a lotion with carrot and rose essential oils	a lotion with lavender essential oil	a lotion with lavender and bergamot essential oils

Three

⋅

Quick Repair
Beauty
Treatments

One advantage of the at-home spa experience is that it's so easy to tailor your treatments to your special needs. Some weekends you may want to revitalize your hair, others you may decide it's time for an hour-long facial. The basic spa programs that we outline in Chapter 10 are designed as templates to guide you. You can include—or leave out—specific treatments, depending on what requires your attention. To help you personalize your spa routine, this chapter targets problem areas and offers a wide selection of treatment options for:

- hair
- elbows
- eyes
- feet
- hands and nails
- thighs

Hair Repair

The health of your hair mirrors the health of your whole body—lack of good nutrition can dull and damage the hair; stress and tension can cause scalp and skin problems. But even those of us who are conscientious about taking care of ourselves can have problem hair that is dry, oily, limp, or just plain out of control. Fortunately, there are many treatments you can use to restore shine and body and make your hair easier to style. Here are a few favorites that you can do at home:

FOR DRY HAIR AND SCALP

If you infuse dry hair and scalp with moisture and oil, you will increase shine, prevent damage to the hair shafts and follicles, and increase manageability. We suggest you begin with a scalp treatment; then apply a conditioner to the hair itself; next wash with a gentle, commercial shampoo; and finally condition with a vitalizing rinse.

You may enjoy giving yourself a hair treatment immediately before taking an aromatic soak (see Chapter 4). That way you can let the hair treatment work while you relax in the tub. If you repeat the following treatment once a month, you'll keep your hair in top condition.

Hot Oil Scalp Treatment

◆

1 large bath towel
1 cup olive oil
1 clean basting or paintbrush at least 2 inches wide

Hair Conditioning

◆

¼ cup mayonnaise
2 tablespoons oil (olive, avocado, or almond)
1 showercap or plastic wrap

Vitalizing After-Shampoo Rinse

◆

4 cups water (springwater is best)
½ cup cider vinegar
½ cup finely chopped fresh mint leaves
(Before you put the hot oil treatment on your hair, chop
the mint leaves and simmer in the water for 2
minutes. Allow to steep and cool while you're doing
the treatment.)

Pour 1 cup olive oil into small saucepan or coffee cup.
Place on low burner or in microwave until hot to touch. Do
not allow to boil, smoke, or scorch.

As the oil is heating, steam a bath towel in hot—but not
boiling—water. Press out extra liquid. Fold into small square
to hold heat until you're ready to use it.

Starting at the center part, section hair into squares about
2 inches long and 2 inches wide. Keeping the brush near the
roots, paint the scalp with the hot olive oil. The oil should
saturate the scalp and hair about 1–2 inches from the scalp.

When scalp is well painted, apply the mayonnaise dry-hair conditioner to the ends of the hair. You may use the basting brush or your fingers. When hair is completely coated, put on shower cap. Then wrap your hair, turban-style, in a hot bath towel.

Slip into a soothing bath, using either the chamomile soak on page 80, or the moisturizing soak on pages 81–83.

After a minimum of 20 minutes, remove towel and rinse hair in lukewarm water. Shampoo hair with a mild formula made especially for dry hair. Towel dry.

To finish your hair treatment, add cider vinegar to lukewarm mint tea. Pour the rinse over hair, removing all soapy residue that can dry scalp and hair. Keep out of eyes.

FOR OILY HAIR AND SCALP

Oily hair can look stringy and lifeless, provoke facial blemishes, and guarantee a bad hair day. But you can bring body and swing to your tresses by using oil-reducing shampoos, shine-enhancing conditioners, and refreshing rinses.

Oil-Reducing Shampoo for Those with Brown, Dark Red, or Black Hair

•

Mild, non-oily shampoo
1 amber beer
1 saucepan

If you have dark-colored hair—boil beer until about half has evaporated. Let cool and mix with about ¼ cup of shampoo.

Wash hair with tepid water.

Rinse for a full 2 minutes with lukewarm water. Repeat.

Oil-Reducing Shampoo for Those with Light-Colored Hair

◆

Mild, non-oily shampoo
2 tablespoons fresh lemon juice
½ fresh lemon peel, as intact and large as possible

If you have light-colored hair, combine ¼ cup shampoo with the juice of 1 lemon. Whisk until blended.

Wash hair in lukewarm water and rinse completely for about 2 minutes. Repeat.

After last rinse, take the lemon rind and rub the inside white coating on your hair. Let sit for about 3 minutes. Rinse again.

Shine-Enhancing Conditioner for All Hair Colors

◆

¼ cup honey or more as needed to coat hair
1 tablespoon hot water

Combine ¼ cup honey with 1 tablespoon hot water. Stir well and apply to hair at roots, then spread toward ends. If you have long hair, use as much honey as you need to condition well. Don't worry, it rinses out. Wrap hair in plastic wrap or a plastic shower cap and then wrap a towel around that. Allow the honey to soak into hair for 5 to 10 minutes. Rinse well in lukewarm water. Pat dry.

Herbal Hair Treatments

Herb-infused oils can be used as conditioners after shampooing. Herb teas can be used as rinses to remove shampoo residue from hair, increase shine, and help repair damaged hair shafts.

For herb infused oils:
- Use about ½ cup fresh herbs or 1 ounce dried herbs for every 2 cups of oil. Place in sterile, airtight glass jar and allow to infuse at room temperature for at least 3 days.
- Strain through a coffee filter before using as conditioner. Store in the refrigerator, but bring to room temperature before using.

For herb teas:
- Use 2–3 teabags or 3 tablespoons loose herbs for every quart of water. Pour boiling water over herbs into sterile container and steep at room temperature for 2 hours.
- Strain and store in the refrigerator, but use as rinse at room temperature.

Herbs to Use

FOR DRY HAIR	FOR OILY HAIR	FOR NORMAL HAIR	FOR MORE SHINE
chamomile	peppermint	fennel	basil
parsley	rosemary	rosewater	parsley
sage	witch hazel	basil	rosemary

Refreshing Rinse for All Hair Colors

◆

juice of one fresh lemon
2 quarts water
1 teaspoon fresh grated ginger root

Combine juice of 1 fresh lemon with 2 quarts warm water. Place ginger inside a coffee filter tightly closed with tape or inside a tea bomb or a piece of nylon stocking. Let ginger steep in the lemon water for 5 minutes. Pour half the mixture over hair, squeeze out, and repeat. Towel dry hair gently.

FOR INCREASED SHINE

One of the tricks that spa therapists use to help restore life to dull, damaged hair is the scalp massage. It stimulates blood flow to the scalp and hair follicles and helps nutrients feed hungry hair shafts. You can duplicate this at home.

First, leaning over the sink so that your blood is flowing toward the scalp, apply the conditioner. Rub it in slowly and thoroughly. Then, if you are comfortable, remain with your head bent forward while you give yourself a scalp massage (or have your spa partner do this). Massage the scalp by squeezing the skin in soft, fat pinches. Do it in a systematic, circular pattern around the entire scalp. Then, using your fingertips, lightly vibrate your fingers against the scalp for two minutes. Here are some recipes for shine-enhancers that are good for any hair type:

Yogurt Egg Elixir

◆

Apply this to freshly shampooed or dry hair.

1 whole egg plus 1 egg yolk
1 small container of whole milk plain yogurt

or, for oily hair,

1 small container of fat-free plain yogurt
1 tablespoon any herb-infused oil (optional)

Beat together eggs and yogurt. For oily hair use fat-free yogurt and eliminate extra egg yolk.

Coat hair at scalp and ends with mixture and pile hair on head.

Cover hair with shower cap. Then wrap in a warm towel (that you've put in the dryer for 5 minutes or steamed with hot water and wrung out).

Let conditioner soak in for 20 minutes.

Rinse in *cool* water. (Hot water can cook the egg—and that's not a mess you want to have to deal with.) Comb out with a wide-toothed comb. Let hair air-dry.

Guacamole

◆

After shampooing, apply this elixir—rich in vitamins A and E—to wet hair.

1 very ripe avocado
2 tablespoons avocado oil (canola oil will do)
1 shower cap

Beat avocado and oil together until creamy.

Spread through hair from scalp to ends.

Cover hair with shower cap. Let sit for 10–15 minutes.

Rinse in lukewarm water. Not recommended for oily hair.

See *salsa plus*, on page 64, for an alternative treatment.

Salsa Plus

◆

If you have oily hair *and* want more shine and body, this recipe works wonders.

> *1 small can low-sodium V-8 juice*
> *½ cucumber peeled and seeded*
> *¼ cup low-fat or no-fat sour cream*
> *1 shower cap*

Combine in blender V-8 juice, cucumber, low-fat or no-fat sour cream.

Spread throughout hair.

Cover hair with plastic wrap or shower cap for 10 minutes. Rinse in lukewarm water. Towel dry.

Sweet Solution

◆

Honey provides nutrition for the hair, smoothes the hair shaft, and heals damage caused by sun and hairspray or gel. Good for all hair types.

> *½–1 cup honey*
> *½ cup apple cider vinegar*
> *1 shower cap or plastic wrap*

Spread honey over hair, particularly on the ends if they are split or flyaway.

Cover with shower cap for 30 minutes

Rinse with vinegar diluted in 1–2 quarts warm water.

Smart Shampoo Techniques

- Don't overshampoo your hair. Use only as much as you need to lather the full head and scalp. Extra will only put unneeded chemicals on your already-tired hair.
- Rinse hair completely after each shampoo with lukewarm to cool water. Hot water exhausts the hair shaft, robs the hair of natural oils, and is less effective in removing shampoo residue.
- Dry hair by gently squeezing it in a clean, absorbent towel.
- Comb hair out using a wide-toothed comb—and blow dry, if you must, at as low a temperature as possible.

Hand and Nail Care

Hands contain more nerves than any other part of the body; they are where we interact with the world on the most visceral level—getting a feel for our environment, expressing ourselves through gestures, writing, painting; using the sense of touch to learn of danger and of bliss. We want to take good care of our hands so they can remain as sensitive and as strong as possible.

Today, however, hands take a different kind of beating than they used to when so many people did hard physical labor at home, in the fields, or on the job. Now the constant tension from using a keyboard is the number one crippler, causing wrinkles; muscle, joint, and tendon stiffness; and chronic pain. The following therapies should provide relaxation as they beautify. Use them in conjunction with the hand massage in Chapter 6.

Good nails are a reflection of good nutrition. If you have nails that spilt easily, get hangnails, are discolored or fragile, that's a sign that you should change your eating habits and consume more pure water. Chances are you need to reduce your fat intake, cut down on caffeine, increase the amount of fruits, leafy green vegetables and beans you eat, and perhaps, stop smoking. These are long-term therapies for the basic health of your hands and nails. But there are many simple treatments that can improve their appearance quickly.

- Coat your hands and nails in honey for 15 minutes once a week to make your skin silky and smooth and to help improve dry, brittle nails.
- Use a mixture of 1 tablespoon fine-ground oatmeal, ½ teaspoon canola oil, and a squirt or two of lemon juice as a hand "soap" to eliminate drying and irritation.
- Soak hand and nails in a milk bath of half-and-half for 20 minutes once a week.
- Apply to your hands suitable facial masks described in the section beginning on page 5 or any of your favorite commercially made masks.
- Even something as simple as breaking open 1 or 2 capsules of vitamin E and spreading the liquid on your cuticles and nails will have a wonderful effect—soothing irritation, softening cuticles, and nurturing the nail bed.

In addition you may enjoy the following special therapies:

Deep Moisturizing
Use this once a week to keep your nails healthy, your skin silky, and to remove toxins.

coconut oil or coconut butter
2 large Baggies
tape
1 heating pad

Wash hands with mild cleanser in warm water and pat dry.

Coat backs of hands, fingers, palms, and nail beds with coconut oil or butter.

Place each hand in a large plastic Baggie and close ends at wrists.

Place on top of preheated heating pad. Cover hands and pad with a towel. (If no heating pad is available, you may place the well-sealed Baggies in a pan of water that is comfortably hot—not warm. Make sure no water seeps into the Baggies.)

Allow oil to soak in for about 7 minutes. We recommend that while you are enjoying the hand treatment you take the opportunity for a 5-minute meditation (see Chapter 7). **Do not combine use of a heating pad with any water-based treatments such as foot soaks or facial steams.** Follow with a hand massage (see page 125 for instructions).

Targeting the Nails

Soak fingertips in warm water with a drop of essential oil or an herb-infused oil (see page 29 for instructions) for 4 minutes. Lavender will soothe your skin, chamomile will soften it, and peppermint (the essential oil form of this herb is not for pregnant women—use peppermint tea) will stimulate circulation.

When you take your hands out of the water, immediately apply a coat of rich cream or oil—such as coconut butter or almond oil—to nails and cuticles. Allow to sit for 5 minutes. Gently rub off excess with cotton balls.

Your Best Foot Forward

According to acupuncturists and reflexologists, you can communicate with many other parts of the body through the foot. For example, reflexologists identify the area along the outer edge of the bottom of the foot, just under the little toe, with the arm—rub that part of the foot and you can help dispel tension that may accumulate from working at a keyboard, for example. And acupuncturists locate the endpoint of many powerful meridians in the feet—needling or massaging those regions can have positive repercussions on the health of internal organs, the mind, and the spirit.

Many spa treatments concentrate on improving the appearance of your feet—but in truth they also take advantage of the healing aspects of working on the feet. When you spend time soaking and creaming and rubbing your feet, you'll find that your whole body responds positively. So jump right in. And when you're done, try a reflexology foot massage (described on pages 124–25).

TO DISPEL TENSION, SOFTEN CALLUSES, AND REMOVE TOXINS

The three treatments offered here should make your feet more beautiful and help dispel stress.

For a Relaxing Soak

◆

½ cup loose chamomile tea
1 large basin

canola oil or moisturizing cream
1 old stocking (optional) and 1 tennis ball

Bring 1 gallon of water to a boil, if possible in a pan that's large enough to use to soak your feet. Add loose chamomile (you may put it in an old stocking, tied tightly, if you don't want it floating around in the water) or 6 teabags and allow to steep for 5 minutes. When water is cool enough for you to put your feet in, soak for at least 10 minutes.

When done, pat dry but leave moist. Rub with oil.

For an effective foot self-massage—sit in a comfortable straight-back chair. Place tennis ball on the floor in front of you. Put the arch of one foot on the ball. Pressing down, roll the ball back and forth across your arch—up to the ball of your foot and down to you heel. Take it slowly, feeling the sensations at each area of your foot. Repeat on other foot.

To Help Remove Calluses

◆

¼ cup Epsom salts
¼ cup baking soda
¼ cup sea salt
3 gallons water
pumice stone
rich foot cream

Boil water in large basin and stir in salts and baking soda. Mix until well dissolved.

When water cools slightly, soak feet for 10–15 minutes. Towel dry and cover with thin coating of foot cream. Use pumice stone on calluses and rough spots.

Soak again for 5 more minutes. Towel dry and coat with heavy moisturizer.

To Cool Swollen, Hot, Tired Feet

◆

4 peppermint tea bags
2 tablespoons rosemary
2 tablespoons thyme or lemon-thyme
1 lemon
1 tray of ice cubes
1 old stocking

Place herbs in a section of old stocking and tie off ends. Steep herbs in ½ gallon boiling water for 10 minutes. Slice lemon into thin rounds and drop in brew.

In basin large enough to soak your feet, add 1 gallon cool water to tea and a tray of ice cubes. Slip your feet into the basin and soak for as long as you like the feeling.

To Soften Skin and Smooth Heels

◆

2 large plastic bags or Baggies
heavy moisturizer cream or coconut butter
masking tape

Boil 1–2 gallons of water in a large basin.

Wash feet in gentle soap and lukewarm water. Pat dry and coat with foot cream or coconut butter.

Place each foot in a Baggie and secure around your ankle with tape.

Soak your Baggie-clad feet in the basin of hot water for ten minutes. Be careful not to let any water into the Baggies.

Remove Baggies and massage feet (see pages 122–25).

3-in-1 Elbow Therapy

Although nothing but vigorous toning exercises (see pages 148–52) can help tighten the droopy skin around an elbow that comes with age, becoming overweight, or lack of physical activity, you can eliminate dry, rough spots. And for the rather homely elbow (it's just how they were made!) that's a big improvement.

Step One: For Softening Compress

♦

2 hand towels
¼ cup loose chamomile tea or 3 tea bags

Step Two: To Remove Dead, Dry Skin

♦

¼ cup granulated sugar
2 tablespoons canola oil

Step Three: To Deep Moisturize

♦

coconut butter, vitamin E oil, or another heavy,
  pure moisturizer
plastic wrap
3 foot-long strips of gauze, cut in half

Brew chamomile tea for 5 minutes. Mix sugar and oil in a small bowl and set aside for later use.

Soak hand towels in tea. Wring out and fold into thirds

lengthwise. Wrap around elbows. Allow elbows to steam for about 5 minutes. Remove towels.

Pick up a large pinch of sugar and oil with your fingers and scrub elbow in a circular motion. You should do this over the sink, since the sugar scatters as you scrub. Repeat for other elbow. You should scrub each elbow twice, for about 10 seconds each time.

Rinse with chamomile tea. Pat dry with towel.

Spread elbow with moisturizer. Wrap gauze around elbow. Cover with a strip of plastic wrap—you will probably want to wrap it around your arm several times. Let elbow skin drink in oil for 10 minutes.

Thigh Smoothers 4-in-1 Therapy

Cellulite disappears only from a combination of frequent, vigorous exercise and a healthy diet, but you can help the body eliminate pockets of fat and you can tone the skin so that it appears smoother if you use the wrap, scrub, tone, and rub techniques described below. You may choose to do any one of them, but they are most effective when done as a series of treatments.

Step One: Purifying Leg Wrap

•

We offer two versions of this wrap: the herbal wrap and the seaweed wrap.

> *1–2 cups dried herbs (rosemary, thyme, basil, sage,*
> *lavender, peppermint, tarragon)*
> *1 plastic sheet, drop cloth (from a hardware store), or old*
> *shower curtain*

1 sheet

2 oversize bath towels

1 basin of very hot, boiling water

or

2–3 ounces kelp powder (available in health food stores)—
use less if you are combining other sea plants, more if
you're not

4 ounces pure aloe vera gel

1 large basin of very hot, not boiling water

1 plastic sheet, drop cloth (from a hardware store), or old 1
sheet shower curtain

2 oversize bath towels

For herbal wrap:

Although you can do this yourself, you might want a partner
for this treatment to help with the wrapping.

Heat water in basin and steep herbs for 5 minutes.

Soak bath towels in herbal tea and wring out until wet
but not dripping.

Place plastic sheet over bed or padded mat, top with a
sheet.

Wrap legs tightly from ankle to hip in herb-soaked bath
towels.

Lie back on mattress and fold sheet tightly around yourself.

Close eyes and breathe deeply and evenly. Lie in darkened
room with soothing music playing for 10 minutes or until the
towels cool. If you are chilled, wear a T-shirt or drape a blanket over your torso.

For kelp wrap:

Although you can do this yourself, you might want a partner
for this treatment to help with the wrapping.

In a basin of hot, not boiling water, mix aloe gel and kelp powder. If you have other sea plants, fresh or dried, you may add in. You can place the seaweed (not the powder) directly on your skin after steeping and then wrap the soaked towels around your legs. Remember to wash off afterward. Remember these plants are very rich in iodine and other nutrients and quite potent. You don't want to use too much. **With herbs *more* and *longer* are not always better.**

Proceed with the wrap as described above.

Step Two: Circulation-Enhancing Scrub

◆

1 cup fine ground raw oatmeal
1 tablespoon vinegar (cider is best)
¼ cup whole milk
2 cups boiling water
1 tablespoon rosemary or fennel

This formula is good for thighs, calves, feet, arms, back, and torso. Remember to do it gently.

In a large bowl combine oatmeal and boiling water. Stir well and let sit for 1 minute. Add milk and vinegar. Let sit for another minute.

While you're waiting, pour about a half cup of water over the rosemary or fennel and let steep for a minute. Add liquid and herbs to the oatmeal mixture. Stir well.

You will probably want to do this standing in an empty tub or shower stall. Soak a washcloth in hot water and apply to legs as hot compress. When legs are cleaned and warmed, take about 2 tablespoons of the oatmeal mixture and place in the center of the washcloth. Use that to rub your outer thighs in small circles starting at the hip and working down toward the knee. Repeat on all areas of the legs.

Rinse legs with lukewarm water and follow with toning splash and moisturizing treatment below.

Step Three: Skin-Toning Splash

◆

¼ cup aloe vera gel
¼ cup witch hazel
¼ cucumber, peeled, seeded, and pureed
fine strainer

This formula is good for thighs, calves, feet, arms, back, and torso.

Combine aloe vera and witch hazel.

Peel and seed a cucumber. Puree in blender. Add to aloe mixture.

Pour liquid through a small-screened sieve.

Chill the liquid in the refrigerator for about 30 minutes.

Apply to thighs by pouring into palm of hand and then gently slapping it onto the skin.

Step Four: Deep Moisturizing Treatment

◆

honey

You may want to do this sitting on the edge of an empty tub, with your feet in the tub.

Slather honey on your thighs, especially where the skin is dimpled or rough. Rub it into the skin vigorously. (Apply honey only to legs that are cleansed and warmed.)

You can wrap the honey-covered thigh in plastic wrap to

increase heat and contact between the honey and your skin. Leave for 10–15 minutes. Wash off with warm water. Pat dry.

Emergency Eye Treatments

The eyes may be the window to the soul, but they're also a billboard informing the passing world about your health and your mood. Tired? The eyes will tell. Sad? Ditto. Angry, worried, strained, happy, gleeful, well exercised? Eating right? There's nothing that the eyes can't reveal about how you're doing. So while we advocate that you eat right, get enough sleep, and avoid excess alcohol and stress, you'll find the following anti-redness and puffiness remedies refreshing and effective.

The skin around the eyes is the most delicate on the body. It's thin, has few oil ducts, and tends to be quite dry. That's why it's important to protect it from exposure to the sun and to treat it gently at all times. You shouldn't scrub around the eyes, and remember to apply all lotions with a cotton ball or your fingertips, using a light patting motion.

To Lessen Redness and Puffiness

◆

2 chamomile tea bags
or
2 slices organic cucumber
or
2 large cotton balls soaked in whole milk

Steep two chamomile tea bags in boiling water for 1 minute. Remove from the cup and press excess liquid out of tea bag.

Place tea bag in freezer for 2 minutes or until lightly chilled.

Lie back on the bed or sofa and relax. Place tea bags over your closed eyes. Rest comfortably for 5–10 minutes. Practice your deep breathing. You may also enjoy a deep-moisturizing hand treatment (see pages 65–67).

or

Slice a cucumber into very thin rounds. Place one or more over each eye as needed to cover entire eye area. Drape eyes with a damp, cool washcloth folded into thirds lengthwise. Rest comfortably for 10 minutes.

or

Soak a sterile cotton ball in whole milk or cream and squeeze out so it is quite moist but not runny. Place cotton balls over eyes, covering the entire eye area. Rest for 10 minutes.

For Dry, Drawn Skin

◆

Vitamin E oil, from capsule or bottle

Pat vitamin E oil onto skin around eye, but keep out of eyes! Use *very* sparingly on upper lid.

The oil is very heavy and sticky so it is not meant for application before going out or going to sleep. Instead, let it soak in for 15 minutes. Then pat off excess gently with cotton ball.

Four

•

Steamy Tubs and Soothing Soaks

Soaks bring deep relaxation to the body and the mind, dispelling tension, influencing your mood with subtle aromas, and replenishing the skin. So, for a most pleasurable interlude, light a scented candle, put on some meditative music, and draw yourself a bath.

Hydrotherapy Basics

This chapter presents four types of soaks: herbal infusions, moisturizers, cleansers, and aromatics. *Herbal infusions* are made by steeping fresh or dried herbs in hot water and then adding the tea to the bath. *Moisturizers* act as humectants that hydrate and protect natural oils in the skin. *Cleansers* remove surface pollutants and help detoxify the body. *Aromatics* are created by using essential oils in a bland oil base (such as canola oil) or mixed with a foaming gel.

Whatever sort of tub or soak you use, remember: **All baths should be between 80° and 100° F. Over 100° F can cause dehydration, burst capillaries, and strip oils from skin.**

Herbal Infusions

Herbal infusions soothe the skin, relax tense muscles, and through inhalation of the aroma, ease the spirit.

Tip: To avoid health hazards and assure the best results, always use pesticide-free herbs for spa treatments.

Below is a description of a chamomile soak. It should serve as a template for all other herbal soaks. If you use fresh herbs—such as peppermint—double the amount recommended in the recipe below and chop them into fine pieces before brewing to release their juices.

For Relaxation

◆

Herbs recognized for their relaxing qualities include:

- lavender
- basil

- chamomile
- valerian

General Supplies You'll Want To Have On Hand

- loofah mitt
- large natural sponge
- pumice stone
- neck pillow
- washcloth
- pair old panty hose

You may use these herbs singly or in combination.

1 cup loose chamomile tea
1 piece of nylon stocking to use as a tea bag
1 large basin of boiling water
1 large natural sponge
1 washcloth
1 neck pillow

Place herbs in length of nylon stocking and tie off the ends.

Place in basin of boiling water. Turn off heat. Allow to steep for 5 minutes. Squeeze liquid from tea bag of herbs. Set aside.

Pour tea into a warm bath.

Dim the lights, light a scented candle, turn on the music, and slip into the soothing waters. Remember to use your neck pillow. Do not use soap or cleansers of any kind.

Soak up spongefuls of the bathwater and squeeze over your entire body; then use the sponge to rub your skin gently, removing dead skin. You may also make a warm compress from the tea water using your washcloth. Soak it in the tea and, with your eyes closed, drape it over your face to gently steam-clean the pores. Lean back on your neck pillow and relax. Soak until water begins to cool.

You may rinse off in warm water.

For Sore Muscles

◆

Follow the instructions for the relaxing chamomile tub above. Use fresh or dried peppermint, fennel, and/or marjoram.

For Exhaustion

◆

Use fresh or dried fennel and/or sage.

For Puffiness or Swollen Feet or Hands

◆

Use fresh or dried peppermint, thyme, and/or basil.

Moisturizing Soaks

For Dry Skin

◆

You'll be as smooth as Cleopatra's asp, if you use her famous milk 'n' honey bath.

2 cups powdered whole milk
8 ounces raw or clover honey
2 tablespoons rosemary tied into a length of nylon stocking

Mix milk with 1 gallon water. Heat on stovetop until hot. Stir in honey and mix well.

Pour into a warm bath. Slip into the tub. Relax using your neck pillow. Soak until water cools.

Rinse off well in warm shower. Towel dry gently.

For Tired Skin

♦

Tired skin lacks moisture, is drawn, and may be ashen or off-color. Although the two simple soaks described below produce quite distinct sensations, they both feed your hungry skin. Vinegar helps restore the skin's acid mantel and prevents loss of natural oils and moisture. Oatmeal nurtures the skin with a rich mix of vitamins and minerals. Once you're done with either one, the best thing you can do is drink plenty of springwater, have a well-balanced low-fat dinner, and get eight hours of sleep.

1 cup cider vinegar
1 cup chopped fresh peppermint and/or rosemary and
    thyme
or
¼ cup dried herbs
1 neck pillow

Boil 2 quarts of water. Add herbs and let seep for 5 minutes. Strain herbs from tea.

Pour cider vinegar into tea.

Add mixture to a hot bath.

Slip in. Don't use any soaps or cleansers. Soak for 10 minutes. Towel dry.

1 cup finely ground oatmeal
2 cups boiling water
½ cup whole milk
1 loofah mitt (not for sensitive skin)

Combine oatmeal, milk, and boiling water. Stir well. Add to shallow, warm bath.

Slip in. Using your loofah mitt, scoop up the oatmeal-laced, milky water and massage your thighs, lower legs, arms, shoulders, and torso. Use a gentle circular motion; don't scrape the skin. If a loofah is too harsh for your skin, use a nylon net buffer or your hands.

Rinse off with warm or cool water. Moisturize with a mild body cream.

You may want to combine the oatmeal soak with an oat-meal moisturizing scrub. Mix together ½ cup thick, in-expensive cold cream, ¼ cup ground oatmeal, and 2–3 tablespoons honey. Use with loofah over whole body while soaking in the oatmeal bath.

Cleansers

You can use a soak to clean your skin of pollutants and to help detoxify your internal organs as well.

For Detoxification

♦

The skin not only acts as a landing strip for airborne pollutants, it is the organ through which many internal toxins pass as they are excreted out of the body. The result is that skin can become clogged—an environmental disaster. Luckily there are natural substances that help purge toxins from the skin. Sea plants such as kelp and salt are among the most effective.

¼ cup kelp powder
½ cup aloe vera gel

Run a warm to hot bath.

Pour kelp powder and aloe gel under the running water to mix well.

Soak in tub for 20 minutes. Shower off in tepid water. Moisturize.

For Deep Cleansing

♦

1 cup sea salt
1 cup Epsom salts
1 cup baking soda
¼ cup coconut butter

Run a warm to hot bath.

Pour salts under running water to dissolve. Add baking soda. Stir well.

Soak for 20 minutes.

Rinse in warm water. Towel dry.

Spread coconut butter all over your skin, concentrating on dry spots.

Aromatics

Aromatherapy is based on essential oils distilled from plants and uses their health-giving properties to remedy physical and emotional travails. Depending on which oil you select, your aromatic bath can help you manage almost anything—from depression to indigestion.

You must, however, use essential oils cautiously. They smell so good that many people forget they are potent medicines with potentially dangerous side effects. (See page 17 for more information on toxicity.)

• Because the oils may cause irritation, it's important not to pour them directly into your bathwater but to add them to some neutral carrier such as canola oil or a bath gel.

• In fact, basil, thyme, ti-tree, peppermint (not for pregnant women), lemon, lemon grass, and lemon verbena essential oils are potentially so irritating that you can use only 2–3 drops, diluted in 3 tablespoons of canola oil, in a whole tub of water. Other potential irritants: thyme (not recommended for anyone with high blood pressure), parsley seed, sweet fennel (not for pregnant women), cinnamon leaf, Siberian fir needle, and pimenta leaf.

To enjoy the benefits and health-giving powers of aromatherapy, follow the guidelines, and buy essential oils only from trained aromatherapists who can instruct you on the nuances of use.

To Increase Passion

¼ cup canola oil (or bath gel)
15 drops ylang-ylang, or
5 drops each of ylang-ylang, peppermint, and/or ginger

(Peppermint essential oil should not be used by pregnant women.)

Mix essential oils with canola oil or bath gel.
Add to a medium-hot bath right before you slip in.
Soak for 20 minutes. Concentrate on your breathing. Allow the aromatics to penetrate your senses.

To Dispel Tension

♦

Use lavender and orange essential oils. Follow instructions above. **Orange essential oil may cause photosensitivity.** Make sure to rinse off well after using in a bath and don't go into the sun with the oil on your skin.

For Sore Muscles

♦

Use rosemary and thyme essential oils. Follow instructions above. **Rosemary should not be used by pregnant women and rosemary and thyme should not be used by anyone with high blood pressure.**

For Tranquillity

♦

Use rosewater in amount needed to achieve a pleasant aroma. Do not use more than ½ cup. Sprinkle water with organic rose petals, if available. **(This is important: If you are unsure if petals are free of pesticides, don't use them!)**

Five

Cocoons of Pleasure: Body Wraps and Scrubs

Body wraps may have originated thousands of years ago in the lands around the Nile where the privileged classes are thought to have coated their skin in scented mud and then covered themselves in soft fabrics to beautify their skin and fend off ill health. Today, such wraps have become a specialized part of the spa experience and many facilities offer exotic treatments using seaweeds, muds, herbs, and oils.

All types of wraps are designed to help beautify your skin by infusing it with moisture and nutrients. But the wraps do much more than that: Being swaddled like a small babe in a warm, soothing cocoon purges muscles of stress and soothes the spirit.

In addition to body wraps, many spas are offering clients all-over body scrubs that stimulate circulation more actively than wraps do. These sybaritic sensations are both invigorating and relaxing—a great way to dispel tension without losing energy.

To create these same therapeutic experiences at home, you can use the recipes given in this chapter or buy any of the prepackaged soaks, scrubs, and masks that are available at body and bath shops. Try these at the end of a long day, as part of your weekend at-home spa routine or with your partner for a sensual interlude.

Body Wrap Basics

♦ Before you have a body treatment, you want to cleanse yourself with a gentle, quick shower or bath using a mild cleansing lotion to remove all makeup, body lotions, perfumes, and surface pollutants.

♦ To create the wrap, you can cover your bed with a plastic sheet, drop cloth, or shower curtain. Place a sheet over it. Once you apply the treatment of your choice, you may lie down on the sheet and wrap it tightly around you—from chin to toe. Then wrap yourself in the plastic sheeting to hold in heat and help the treatment work more effectively.

♦ Those of you who don't have a setup that allows you to comfortably or neatly wrap up in your bedroom or outside on a patio might consider wrapping in the bathroom and then—with a pillow for your head and neck and a cotton blanket or bath towel to lie on—stretching out in the empty tub for the duration.

♦ If you do this, we recommend that you run a hot shower for a couple of minutes before lying in the tub. This warms the tub and the air in the room so that you don't get a chill and are in a well-humidified atmosphere.

◆ To increase the effectiveness of the wraps—and to stay warm longer—after you wrap yourself in the infused sheet, you may wrap yourself in a plastic drop cloth or plastic wrap. If you don't use the plastic overwrap, you may need a cotton blanket or heavy terry-cloth robe to put over the wrapping to keep from becoming chilled.

◆ Want to maximize your treatment time while you are letting the wrap do its wonderful work? You can combine a wrap with a facial if you want, but it always seems like too much to get together at one time. Better to relax and enjoy each treatment separately. A more restful use of the time is to practice your breathing and meditation.

◆ After every wrap, drink at least 16 ounces of spring-water.

For Deep Moisturizing and Softening

The Avocado Oatmeal Mud Wrap

◆

You can buy ready-to-mix mud formulas at your local body and bath shop, but this homemade mud substitute produces glowing, supple skin as well.

> 1 sheet (use a twin if that will wrap you up snugly
> and completely, with plenty of overlap, otherwise
> use a full-size)
> 1 plastic bag

3–4 ripe avocados
1 cup olive or almond oil (canola oil will do, too)
2 cups oatmeal
springwater (if needed to achieve right consistency)
plastic wrap or a plastic drop cloth

Grind the oatmeal to a fine grain in the blender. Peel avocado and place meat in blender with oats. Add oil, then water, slowly until you have a blended paste. You may not use all of the oil.

At the same time place a bedsheet in a pot of hot but not boiling water. Wring out and fold into a tight square. Place in plastic bag and close.

Take mixture and bag containing the sheet into bathroom. Run hot water in the shower for several minutes to heat tub and air. Turn off water and place bath towel on bottom of tub and arrange pillow for your neck.

Standing on the towel in the tub, spread the avocado mixture over your body—targeting the breasts, thighs, buttocks, and upper arms.

Wrap hot sheet tightly around your body from ankles to chin. Top with plastic wrapper or terry-cloth robe.

Lie down in warmed tub. Allow "mud" to seep into your skin for 15 minutes or until the sheet cools. You don't want to become chilled.

Rinse off in tepid water, using a brisk circular motion to gently scrub the skin as you remove the treatment.

The Milk and Honey Wrap

◆

This adaptation of the famous milk 'n' honey bath (see page 81–82) leaves you relaxed and calm and your skin soft and well nourished.

1 sheet (*use a twin if that will wrap you up snugly and
    completely, with plenty of overlap*)
powdered whole (not low- or nonfat) milk
*raw honey without the comb, or, if not available, standard
    clover honey*
water

In a large lobster pot or basin mix up 2 gallons of powdered milk using hot but not quite boiling water. Add ½ cup
more dry milk than the instructions call for. Stir well.

Pour at least 1 cup of honey into hot milk. Stir well.

Put a sheet in the mixture. Cover pot to retain heat. Allow
to soak for at least 3 minutes.

Bring pot with sheet and one jar of honey—it's safest and
most convenient if you use a plastic squeeze bottle—into the
bathroom.

Warm the tub and the air by running the hot shower.
Turn off shower and place the bath towel lengthwise in the
tub and arrange the pillow for your head and neck.

Squeeze honey all over your body, and spread it around
with your hands, coating yourself thoroughly.

Remove hot sheet from pot and wring out extra liquid.
Wrap tightly around your body from ankles to chin. Top with
plastic wrapper or terry-cloth robe.

Recline in warmed tub for at least 20 minutes, or until
sheet cools. Do not allow yourself to become chilled.

For Energizing and Stimulating

Sometimes you want to use an herbal wrap to stimulate
circulation and invigorate your body and your senses. This
is particularly good if you're tired or stressed but cannot

escape the current demands of your schedule. Using this rosemary wrap lets you retire to your corner between rounds and then get back out in the ring and put up a good fight once again.

The Rosemary Oil Wrap

◆

Rosemary is invigorating but you may also use peppermint, fennel, and/or sage.

> 1 sheet (use a twin if that will wrap you up snugly and
>   completely, with plenty of overlap)
> 1 stocking
> ½ cup dried rosemary or
> 2 cups fresh rosemary or
> a combination of 3 tablespoons each dried rosemary, fennel,
>   and/or peppermint
> ¼ cup canola oil

In the leg of an old stocking place the herb(s) and tie off both ends.

In a large lobster pot or basin heat water to hot but not boiling and brew a tea using the herb package. Steep for at least 10 minutes. Add oil.

Place flat sheet in pot and allow to steep for 5 minutes. Stir occasionally.

In bathroom, with tub prepared as described above, wrap yourself tightly in the hot sheet and top with plastic wrapper or terry-cloth robe.

Lie down for 10–15 minutes. Breathe in the aroma of the herbs deeply as you lie with your eyes closed. Don't allow yourself to become chilled.

Rinse off with cool water.

Citrus Spritz

◆

This wrap may sting any little cuts on your body—but it makes you feel so fresh and alive, it's worth it.

> ½ gallon orange juice
> 1 bottle cider vinegar
> 1–2 gallons water
> 1 handful fresh peppermint (optional)

Combine ingredients in large lobster pot or basin. Add sheet and stir well. Heat liquid and sheet. (If basin isn't large enough to heat liquid with sheet on stove top, combine ingredients and sheet in sink. Boil water on stove. Pour into sink and stir. Allow to steep for 5 minutes.)

Drain cloth of excess liquid and wrap tightly around body. Top with plastic wrapper or terry robe.

Recline in padded tub with pillow for head. Relax for 15 minutes or until cloth becomes cool.

Rinse in tepid water. Pat dry.

The Calming Aromatherapy Wrap

◆

Using essential oils such as orange, chamomile and lavender, you can transform your nervous energy into tranquil meditative thought.

> 12 drops essential oil of lavender, orange, and/or chamomile
> 1 spray bottle with 1–1½ cups of water in it
> 1 oversize bath towel

> *1 sheet of plastic, a couple of large plastic bags cut open so*
> *they lie flat, or a plastic drop cloth*
> *1 sheet*

Put on some completely relaxing music and dim the lights.

Shower in warm water using nonsoap cleanser and rinse well. Towel dry.

Add the essential oil(s) to the water bottle.

Spray the towel thoroughly with the scented water.

Wrap the towel around your body.

Place the sheet on the bed. Cover with the plastic.

Lie down on the center of the plastic. Wrap it around you and then cover yourself snugly with the sheet.

Lie back in the dim room and let your eyes fall closed. Concentrate on your breathing. Take in the aroma of the wrap with every inhalation. Imagine it relaxing your body as it spreads out through the muscles.

After 10–15 minutes, take another warm shower, using only the gentlest cleanser. Towel dry.

The Salt Scrub

•

Another all-body treatment that is cleansing and invigorating is the salt scrub. It removes dry skin without causing dehydration. Not for skin with blemishes, irritation, or open cuts. Do not use on face or other delicate areas.

> *1–2 cups sea salt or any other coarse-grained salt*
> *½ as much oil as salt (1 cup salt to ½ cup oil). Use a rich*
> *oil such as almond or coconut.*
> *1 washcloth or scrubbing mitt*

Mix salt with oil until well blended.

Coat entire body with salt-oil mixture. Start with upper arms and shoulders; don't neglect back or buttocks and finish at ankles.

Next, using a washcloth or mitt, massage the salt-oil mixture, ever so gently, into the skin. Always use a gentle circular motion—that relaxes muscles as it treats the skin.

Rinse in tepid shower without soap or any cleanser. Towel dry gently, patting not rubbing.

The Sugar Scrub

♦

Provides a milder all-over scrub than the salt. For any skin type.

2 cups granulated sugar
½ cup canola oil

Mix sugar and oil to form a smooth, thick paste. Add more oil if needed.

Moisten skin by taking a quick, warm shower. Do not dry off.

Dip fingers into sugar mixture and massage all over body—paying special attention to thighs, arms, torso, and feet.

Rinse off in warm shower. Pat dry.

The Healing Touch: Massage Basics

Massage takes you into the realm of the senses where mind and body are joined on a primeval level and there is no boundary between the physical and the spiritual. Touch—in and of itself—is healing, offering comfort and connection, emotional release and stress reduction. The use of specific therapeutic massage techniques offered at spas only amplifies the glorious feelings that come from touch. You have the choice of traditional styles, such as long-stroke Swedish massage and shiatsu, and alternative practices, such as craniosacral touch therapy, reiki, and spinal release massage. But no matter where you go for a massage or what technique is used, the setting is always tranquil and dimly lit, sparklingly clean, with a comfortable table to lie upon, in a room that is warm and often filled with aromatic scents and soothing music. The environment helps you become more receptive to the healing powers of massage.

Even though you don't have the same facilities as a spa, you can do a great deal to recreate this spa atmosphere, which is such a vital part of the therapeutic massage. And while you may not be able to emulate all the techniques used by massage therapists, you will be surprised at how quickly you can master some of their art by following the simple instructions in this chapter. So prepare yourself and your partner for one of the most important health-giving aspects of the total spa experience.

Massage Basics

Creating a spalike massage at home doesn't take a lot of expensive equipment and supplies—but a few great "helpers" can make the whole experience a sybaritic delight. You can make some of the supplies yourself, but they are all available, ready-made, at bath and beauty stores.

Setting the Stage

You'll want to have on hand a bedsheet, four large bath towels (three to make a hot compress and one to drape over the person receiving the massage), a small pillow, an hour-long tape of unobtrusive, restful music, a candle (scented if you wish), a firm bed or table (preferably at a height that won't give the person doing the massage a backache), or, for massaging on the floor, an exercise pad or several blankets covered with a large sheet. And be sure the area is large enough for the person receiving the massage to lie comfortably and for the other person to move around freely. If you are giving the massage, you will want to kneel on the soft surface so your knees don't get sore. (The best position is to kneel on one knee and keep the other leg bent. Then you can lean into the massage, applying pressure with the weight of your body, instead of your hands and fingers. It will keep you from getting exhausted and offers a much smoother, deeper pressure.) If you are giving a seated massage or a self-massage, use a straight-back chair with a lightly padded seat. Remember, the massage oil can stain.

Hot Compresses

Every massage should begin with a five- to ten-minute treatment with a soothing compress. Not only does the damp heat soothe the spirit, warm the muscles, and ease pain, it helps keep the person who's getting the massage from becoming chilled. You can make one from hot, damp towels or use one of the premade compresses listed below.

♦ The towel compress can be made with steamy hot water and a plastic bag.

1. Soak one large bath towel in water that is hot but not quite boiling (or it will be too hot to work with).
2. Wring out so that it is hot and damp but not drippy. Fold in half twice.
3. Repeat with second towel. Place towels in a kitchen garbage bag and fold over, forming a flat, tightly sealed package.
4. If the person receiving the massage is having her back rubbed first, have her lie facedown in the center of a double sheet on a firm mattress or on a mat on the

floor. You may place a small pillow under the hip bones, and for large-breasted women, under the collarbone.

If the person is receiving a massage on the front of her torso, have her recline on her back. Place a small pillow under her knees.

5. Drape one large bath towel lengthwise over the torso—front or back, as appropriate. Place the plastic bag with the towels in it on the torso. Bring the sides of the sheet up over the person so she is well covered from chin to toe and comfortably warm.

6. Allow her to rest for 5–10 minutes, listening to the music, enjoying a scented candle, becoming relaxed.

7. When you remove the compress, if the bath towel covering the person is damp, replace it immediately with a dry one to avoid chilling.

♦ The hydroculator, a premade clay-filled compress, is made to be simmered in a pot of water and then wrapped in a towel before it's placed on the body.

Have the person receiving the massage recline on the sheet. Place a pillow under the knees or hip bones to ease lower back strain and drape the torso with a bath towel. The towel-wrapped hydroculator is then placed on the center of the torso. Wrap the person in the sheet from chin to toe, making sure she is comfortably warm.

Remember to store the hydroculator in the freezer when you are done using it so it won't mildew.

♦ The NecCradel is a shaped tube of grainy material that can be heated up in the microwave and draped over the neck, shoulders, or any body part. It molds to your body shape and retains heat for a long time. For someone with a sore neck or shoulders, start the massage by having the person rest on the

Cradel for 5 minutes. Then begin the head, face, and neck massage described on pages 115–119.

Massage Oils

Massage oil is used to help your hands glide smoothly over the skin. It also increases your sensitivity to muscle texture so you can find tense spots and gauge how much pressure to apply. In addition, the oils moisturize the skin of the person receiving the massage, and when they are scented with essential oils, they can provide aromatherapy.

♦ All oils should be derived from plants, not mineral- or animal-based, and be cold pressed and organic. Canola oil straight from the kitchen cupboard is the best for the least cost—it's light, absorbs well, and makes the skin silky smooth. Almond is also a favorite. The heavier vegetable oils, such as coconut, olive, and avocado, suit some people, but are too oily for most. Peanut oil can trigger allergic reactions. Coconut butter is wonderfully moisturizing, but is best used in small areas, targeting dry patches.

Herb-infused oils add the power of aromatics and herbs to the massage process. Although scented oils are now available at most stores that specialize in bath and beauty products, you can make your own. Use canola or almond oil as the base. Follow the recipes given below. (Remember to store scented oil in the refrigerator but to use only at room temperature.)

lavender/lemon balm for sore muscles
chamomile queller for calmness
rosehips/almond oil rub for sensuality
basil rub for energy

To 1 cup of canola oil add ½ cup (tightly packed) finely chopped, fresh herbs.

Or, if dried herbs are used, crush 3 tablespoons to a fine grain.

Seal or cover the oil. Allow to steep at room temperature for two hours. Then, if you have a blender, blend on puree setting until well mixed.

Strain through a coffee filter or strainer to remove herbs from oil.

Store in refrigerator in a plastic bottle with a tight cap.

Tip: For aromatic massage using essential oils, stick with the more soothing ones such as chamomile or orange with a drop or two of ylang-ylang. Use about 15–20 drops to a ¼ cup of canola oil. Never use essential oils straight on skin! For more information on aromatherapy (including toxicity warnings) see page 17.

Massage Tools

The market is flooded with all kinds of massage tools—electric and hand-powered. Personal taste dictates what you'll enjoy, but some of our favorites include the good old tennis ball, the textured wooden back roller, and the hand-held electric Thumper.

The tennis ball works wonders on tight shoulder or back. Place the ball on the floor and lie down on top of it, avoiding your spine or other bones. For tight leg muscles adjust the position of the ball so that it is pressing directly on the knot.

Relax over it. You may want to stay in that position for up to three minutes at a time.

As for hand-held devices you see in the stores—don't hesitate to try them out, but remember, particularly with the hard wooden tools, *do not press directly on the spine or on any bones.*

The Thumper can be obtained from Wellness America (see resource section on page 230) and is available in a small model that can be used with one hand, making it good for self-massage. This device works by vibrating tense muscles to the point of release. It's effective on the feet as well as the legs and back, but limit exposure to one minute per foot, then switch to the other foot.

For less expensive, but equally relaxing, devices, visit your local drugstore or discount chain or check out the other mail order spa equipment catalogs listed in the resource section.

The Easy Touch

Once you have assembled your basic supplies, it's time to turn your attention to the actual art of using your hands for healing.

A good massage is built on communication between the hands of the person giving the massage and the body of the person receiving it. You don't need to be big and powerful—what's required is gentle, direct effort.

- How you touch is important. So stay relaxed during a massage so you can receive the messages from the muscles.
- Don't press too hard; don't strain yourself.
- Don't massage with half a mind to the task or with a kind of careless disregard—you'll only succeed in making both you and your partner feel worse instead of better.

Your contribution to the healing effect of a massage comes through the *intention* of your touch. That means that when you put your hands on a body you want to be focused on *how* and *why* you are going to touch. For example, when you are starting out, you may think, I want to warm the body and move the tension out of the body. That gives you two action verbs—warm and move—to concentrate on; two objectives to strive for. According to massage therapist Chris Hanckel, L.M.T., the next step is to place yourself in a semi-meditative state that is attuned to the energy of the body you are massaging. That way, when your hands feel a knot or a tense spot on a muscle, you will be able to imagine that knot melting away. Your hands will apply smooth, even pressure against that knot and it will give way.

If all this sounds a little elusive, the results are quite practical. Not only does concentrating on intention allow the person getting the massage to reap the most benefit, it also helps the person giving the massage. You'll find you can move more efficiently and not wear yourself out when your actions are targeted in this way.

Tip: Never massage a person in the area of varicose veins or who has a fever, a contagious disease, a heart condition, or other serious medical problem; is pregnant (unless you are specially trained); or has inflamed joints or large bruises or other skin conditions.

Practicing the Touch

♦ Have the person receiving the massage lie comfortably on her stomach. To make the person more comfortable, you may place a small pillow under the shoulders to lift the torso and make it easier to turn the head to the side; under the hips to ease low back strain; and under the ankles to take pressure off the knees. Experiment to see which combination makes your partner most comfortable. Women with large breasts may be more comfortable with a small pillow under their upper chest.

♦ As the one giving the massage, sit or stand quietly for about 30 seconds, concentrating on your breath. Let your shoulders, arms, and hands fall, gently and relaxed, at your side. Rotate your head from side to side to loosen your neck. Breathe deeply and evenly.

♦ Now place 1 teaspoon of massage oil in the palm of your left hand. (It should make a pool about the size of a quarter.) Rub your two hands together so the oil is evenly distributed and warmed.

♦ Place your hands alongside each other about 1 inch above the surface of the right shoulder blade. Close your eyes. Feel the warmth between your palms and the skin below. Gently lower your hands onto the skin surface and move them in small circles, coating the skin with oil. Expand the circle ever outward until the entire shoulder is lightly oiled. Remember to keep your hands relaxed and in full contact with the muscle.

♦ As you are rubbing, feel the texture of the skin and of the muscles below the skin. Allow your hands to glide, reading the topography of the shoulder.

♦ When you get the feeling of where the areas of tightness are located in the shoulder area, touch the spot with your fingertips. Slowly, moving in circular motions, press down and out around the spot.

Now you can apply your *intention*—to warm and move the area of tension. Using the rubbing techniques explained below, you may warm the skin, and then press through the knot and imagine it melting away like a softened pat of butter. As it melts, you can use your hands to dispel it. You will feel the tension evaporating from that area.

This is the basic way you will use your hands in massage.

Applying the Touch

There are six types of massage strokes that you can use to great effect. Always use a tablespoon of massage oil—rubbed into your hands and then spread over the area to be massaged—before beginning any of the following methods.

- stroking
- kneading
- rubbing or friction
- shaking or trembling
- tapping
- joint movements

Stroking is done over large surfaces—the back, the legs—by gliding the palms of the hands in long strokes over the length of the body. The pressure should be toward the heart—from the feet up; from the shoulders, neck, and head, down; from the wrists toward the shoulders. Over smaller areas—the hands or feet, or one particular area on the back—stroking is done with the fingertips or thumbs.

For example, if you are rubbing the back of the legs, start by the ankle with your hands open and lying flat. Place them lightly on the skin, next to each other with your fingertips pointing up the leg, the heels of your hands at the ankle.

Move both hands together toward the buttocks in a long,

even motion. At first rub up the leg quickly, covering the length of the leg in 2 seconds. Apply smooth pressure as you move your hands up the leg—being careful not to press behind the knee—and then lightly glide your hands back down the leg to the ankle. Repeat, moving hands more slowly, but still using the same long, smooth strokes. (You may repeat the same form along the back and arms.)

Kneading is done with one or both hands and can include grabbing firmly onto a muscle and squeezing while rolling the hands, as you would knead bread. You can also knead with your thumbs or a thumb and finger.

Rubbing, or friction, is different from kneading in that you don't squeeze the skin—you either move your hands across the surface of the skin or keep them planted on one spot but move the muscle under the skin back and forth. You can do this in a circular pattern, using your two hands in unison, or by moving them in opposite directions back and forth across the skin.

You may also use friction to warm an area by placing your palms together in the prayer position, then lowering them so that the outside of each, along the little finger, is about one-half to one-quarter inch above the surface of the skin of the person receiving the massage. Now, rub your palms together vigorously until they become heated—the person receiving the massage will feel the heat and it will help dispel tension and loosen tight muscles. When you're done rubbing your hands, place the warmed palms on the skin surface.

Shaking is the gentle rocking of whole body areas, such as the torso, calves, or upper arms, by using two hands in an even rhythm. The faster version—called vibration—uses hands or fingertips—moving very rapidly over an area in a trembling motion for at least a minute at a time.

Tapping is done by rapidly striking the body with the side of the hands, the fingertips, or a cupped hand. When done for 1 to 10 seconds, it stimulates the muscles. When done for 10 to 60 seconds, it relaxes them. You probably want to limit it to 60 seconds in one spot. And avoid doing this over any area where the muscle is in spasm or highly sensitive.

Joint movements are done two ways—actively, so that the person receiving the massage performs the movements without the help of the person giving the massage; and passively, so that the person giving the massage moves the joint with no help from the other person. Both types are used for stretching muscles and loosening joints. A typical motion is to have the person lie on her back and then bring her knee to the chest. This can be done actively, or the massage therapist can move the leg into that position.

The Full Body Massage

What follows are the instructions for a 40-minute full-body massage. However, it's broken down into various sections of the body—the back, neck, head, torso, legs, and feet. You can do any one or more of those sections by themselves.

Step One: Getting Started

When it comes time to do a massage, you want to choose a location that is comfortable for the recipient and for you as the masseuse—if the surface is too low, or awkward to get around, you'll quickly tire and get a sore back or knees.

♦ Have your partner take off all clothing—except underwear, if that is more comfortable—and then lie down on his or her stomach with a small pillow under the upper chest, knees, and/or ankles. Cover with a clean sheet. The person giving the massage should be in comfortable clothing that

The Effect of Massage

On the skin
- increases healthy flow of skin oils
- sloughs off dead skin cells
- improves oxygenation of skin
- stimulates sweat glands

On muscle tissue
- helps rid the muscles of lactic acid and other waste products that increase muscle fatigue and soreness
- reduces soreness and strain
- helps keep muscles relaxed and stretched so they are at their most efficient and powerful

On circulatory system
- accelerates circulation though vascular and lymph system
- helps reduce blood pressure through relaxation

On nervous system
- may relieve pinched nerves and sedate nervous system
- allows more unimpeded flow of energy through neural network

doesn't bind and that can be easily washed if it becomes stained with massage oil. Choose a firm bed or a tabletop (cushioned with a blanket) that is at a comfortable height for the person giving the massage. You can also give massages on

Seated Massage

If you are more comfortable receiving a massage while you are seated, or giving a massage to a person who is sitting up, you can adopt the techniques described above.

- If you're receiving the massage, you can place pillows on a table so they cushion the edge of the surface and then, seated in a comfortable chair, lean into them. Or you may sit in an upright position, straddling a chair so you're facing the chair back, which is cushioned with a pillow along the back and over the top edge.
- Always support the neck and head.
- When doing leg massages, elevate foot about 4–6 inches off the floor using two phone books or a small footstool.

the floor: Use an exercise mat or several blankets as a cushion. The person giving the massage may want to kneel on a small pillow.

- Dim the lights and play soothing music. Light a scented candle if you wish.

Step Two: The Back

- Have the person stretch out on her stomach. Place another small pillow under her upper chest to make it more comfortable to turn the head to the side. Cover the person from ankles to lower back with a sheet or oversize towel.

Circulation Stimulation and Compression

♦ Keep the person's back covered with the towel. Stand to one side.

Place hands next to each other. Beginning at the small of the back on the side of the spine closest to you, press down on the back (not the spine) with the palms of your hands. The pressure should be toward the feet. Lean onto your hands for the count of three. Release gently. Move hands one hand's width and reapply pressure straight down to table. Put your body weight over your hands and press down (not too hard, let the person tell you what feels good!). Use your body weight to ease the job of massaging. It will help you keep your energy level high.

Continue this rocking motion until you reach the top of the back. Place a hand on either side of the neck with fingers pointing up toward the head. Apply even pressure for the count of three and release. Repeat three times.

♦ Now walk to the other side of the person and repeat the motion going down that side of the spine from shoulder to small of back.

Repeat cycle.

The Upper Back

♦ Move the towel so the back is exposed to the small of the back.

♦ Place 1 tablespoon of massage oil in your palm and rub your hands together to warm the oil. Then smooth it over the entire back and sides of the torso.

♦ Stand above the head, place your palms along the shoulder blades on either side of the spine. With fingers pointing down toward the feet, apply smooth, even pressure to tips, palm, and heel of hand, stretching forward in a gliding motion until the heels of your hands are resting on the tailbone and then moving out along the side of the hips. Gently slide hands up the sides of the body. Keep your hands and fingers relaxed as you rub.

Repeat.

♦ Place hands on the outside of the shoulders, gently squeezing the muscles between the thumb and fingers. Continuing to squeeze and release the muscles, move hands along the edge of the shoulder, toward the top of the spine.

♦ When your hands are at the top of the spine, place your thumbs on either side of the spine and glide them down the length of the spine, applying a steady, even pressure all the way to the small of the back.

♦ Return the thumbs up the back alongside the spine by moving them in a circular motion. Slowly, with pressure, circle them up to the top of the spine.

Repeat three times.

The Shoulder and Back of Arm Rub

♦ Return to the top of the back. Stand at the shoulder. Place both hands on one shoulder. Using the kneading motion of gently squeezing the muscles between the thumbs and fingers, move hands down from the shoulder to the biceps, continuing the length of the arm to the hand. Return to the top of the arm with a smooth gliding motion.

The Side Torso Friction

♦ Stand to one side of the person, even with the lower back. Re-oil your hands and place them palms down along the far side of the torso, fingertips facing toward the far side.

♦ Slowly begin to move the hands in alternating motions back and forth across the side of the torso—when the left one moves toward you, the right one moves away from you. Keep your palms in contact with the skin at all times. This should produce a warming sensation. Move hands up and down the back while moving back and forth. Repeat three times.

Repeat the shoulder arm rub and side friction for the second arm and other side of torso.

The Back Finishing Touch

♦ To complete a back massage, return to standing at the head of the person. Apply ½ tablespoon massage oil to your hands. Using your palms, glide down the length of the back alongside the spine to the small of the back, applying an even, smooth pressure. Glide back up to the shoulders.

Repeat twice.

Step Three: The Back of Legs

♦ Massage the legs from foot to buttocks, using the strongest gliding strokes, moving toward the lower back. Return toward the foot using a feathering technique—moving the fingertips rapidly down the leg as if you were playing an up-tempo piano piece.

♦ Repeat the circulation and compression technique (see page 110) along the length of each leg—pressing for a count of three, releasing, and repeating as you move up the leg. Make sure you **apply no pressure to the back of the knee.**

♦ Spread lotion on hands.

♦ Starting at the heel of the right leg, grab the heel with your full hand and massage deeply. Concentrate on working with the thumb and finger on the area around the Achilles tendon.

♦ Add oil to hands and coat entire leg in oil. Massage the whole length of the leg: Your inside hand glides along the top (with the thumb) and the inside (with the fingers) of the

Lower Back Self-Massage

- Sit on a padded, straight-backed chair. Keep your feet a few inches apart and flat on the floor. Breathe in deeply. Fill up your lungs from the bottom up.

- Exhale, as you lower your chin to your chest. Let your shoulders slump forward and curve your upper back.

- Inhale and continue bending forward, curving your back, keeping your chin at your chest.

- When you are as low as you can go without any strain, rest. Breathe gently.

- Place your hands behind your back and form fists.

- Use your fists to apply pressure in circular pattern to your lower back area. Press along either side of the spine, moving your hands up and down. Pummel your outer hips and upper buttocks.

- Let your arms and hands hang down, limp, at your sides.

- Slowly roll back up, keeping your chin tucked into your chest and your shoulders rounded. Once you are sitting upright, roll up head, neck, and shoulders.

leg, while your outside hand glides along the top (with thumb) and outside (with fingers) all the way on to the buttocks. **Remember—no pressure as you pass over the back of the knee.** Keep strokes long, steady, and smooth.

Repeat three to five times.

♦ Standing at the person's foot, gently lift the foot at the ankle and move the heel toward the buttocks. Do not press—let the person tell you what is comfortable. Rest the foot and shin against your torso and shoulder.

♦ Make sure calf is well oiled. Then, using your thumbs (they will be pointing down) knead the calf from ankle to back of knee. If you find any knots in the muscle, work them gently. Press through, not onto, the knot. Keep thumb motion fluid, not poking. Glide hand back to the heel.

Repeat motion along outside of calf; then along inside. Finish with return to the center.

Repeat entire sequence.

Lay the leg gently back on the massage table.

♦ Starting above the back of the knee, use your thumbs—moving in a circular motion—to rub up the middle back of the thigh. Repeat motion along inside and outside of thigh. (*Tip:* Tuck fingers under hand along inside of thigh.) Now, standing to the side of the person, place the well-oiled palms of your hands next to each other across the thigh. (Your fingertips are curved around the inside of the thigh.) Begin sliding your palms back and forth across the thigh—when one hand goes forward the other goes back. This should create a warmth from the slight friction. Now move your hands back and forth as you go up and down the thigh from knee to buttocks. Press firmly.

♦ Return to the long strokes moving up the leg using both hands. When you reach the top of the leg, return down the leg using a feathering technique. Repeat the stroke up and feathering down three times.

Repeat the entire procedure on the other leg.

Step Four: The Neck

- Have the person flip over onto her back. Place a pillow under the knees to ease lower back tension. Make sure the person is comfortable and warm. Cover with sheet from upper torso to knees or feet, depending on warmth of the room.

- Pour about 1 teaspoon of massage oil into your hands and rub palms together to warm.

- Stand at the head of the person. Place your hands over the shoulders with fingertips facing toward the feet.

- Move hands outward, over and around shoulders.

- Bring them around to the back, under the shoulder blades, so they are between the person's back and the table with the fingers pointing down the back.

- Using a kneading motion squeeze the muscles to the right and left of the spine between your fingers and thumbs. Pulse in and out to work these muscles and loosen them up.

- Then slide your fingers along either side of the spine and, using pressure in your fingertips, slide your hands upward from the shoulder blades, along the neck toward the base of skull. Do not rub directly on the spine.

- Repeat the kneading and gliding up alongside the spine and neck.
Pause.

- Take the person's head in both hands and gently turn to the left. Let rest on table.

- (Make sure your hand is well oiled.) Take the flat of your right palm and rest it along the lower jawbone with the heel of your right hand at the chin and your fingers pointing up to the ear.

- Glide your hand (using a gentle, firm pressure) from the lower jaw to the neck and then angle it downward so the fingertips automatically slide down the back of the neck to the top of the shoulders. **Do not apply any pressure to the front or the sides of neck where the carotid artery is located!**

♦ Glide hands back up to position along jawbone and repeat, turning the head to the right.

Pause

♦ Standing at the person's head, facing her feet, cradle the head in your forearms and cupped palms. Lift the head gently toward the chest. Have the person inhale as you lift the head and exhale as you apply *ever so little* pressure as you bend the chin toward the chest. Hold there for the count of five.

♦ Gently let the head fall back into the cradle of your hands and return it to the tabletop.

Repeat.

♦ Shake off your hands. Let the person rest quietly for a couple of minutes.

Step Five: The Head

♦ Place your hands under the head so that your fingertips are resting at the base of the skull where the head joins the neck. Raise the head up off the table an inch or so and let the full weight of the skull along that ridge fall on your fingertips.

♦ Urge the person to relax fully and let the full weight of the head fall back into your hands. The neck should arch slightly.

♦ Gently pulse your fingers into the bony ridge of the skull without losing contact with the surface.

♦ Now work your way up the back of the head using small circular motions with your fingers. Press up firmly but gently so that you move the scalp and the muscles underneath, not just the hair. Slowly let the head rest back on the tabletop.

♦ Repeat this circular motion over the entire scalp, up onto the forehead and around the ears.

♦ Scratch the entire scalp with your fingertips as if giving a shampoo.

♦ When done, gently pull the hair. Gently.

For self-massage, *you may adopt the suggested motions to your comfort level and ease of execution. A head self-massage combined with the next step—a face and neck self-massage—is an effective way to ease tension and clear the mind so you can relax both body and spirit. Use it before giving yourself a facial.*

Step Six: The Face and Ears

♦ Apply 1 tablespoon pleasant-smelling lotion to your hands and rub palms together to warm. Always use a gentle lotion, instead of oil, when massaging face and ears. Remain standing facing the top of the head, looking down the body.

♦ Place your palms together in a prayer position and put the joined heels of your hands at the chin, with your fingers pointing down the chest and your forearms along the sides of the face. Slowly and evenly part the hands, drawing each one up along the jaw toward the temple, using the palms of the hands to smooth and massage.

♦ Move fingertips to temples and rub gently *around*— not on—the temples.

◆ Place the tips of your index fingers on the inside of the eyes at the bridge of the nose. Apply gentle pressure to the bridge of the nose and move upward toward the eyebrow. Hold that point for 3 seconds. Move outward about the width of your thumb and apply pressure again. Continue this to the outside corner of the eyebrow—then move back to the bridge of the nose and repeat. This is great for people with sinus problems.

◆ Do the same along the bony ridge of the lower eye socket—but be even more gentle.

◆ Starting with the bridge of the nose, trace the thumbs down the nose and across the cheekbones. Use fingertips from the outside edge of the nostrils along lower end of the cheekbones (where they come out of the jawbone). Trace along this jawline to the jaw joint just in front of the ears. Use fairly firm pressure in a circular motion at the jawbone.

◆ Place thumbs under the nose, along the upper lip, and draw them out slowly toward the lower edge of the cheekbones. Repeat. Now move to under the lower lip. Place thumbs in the center of the chin and slowly spread them out toward the jaw joint. Circle your thumbs around the jaw joint.

◆ Starting at the chin put thumbs on top of the lower jaw and fingers under the lower jaw. Pull hands toward ears.

◆ Take ears between index finger and thumb and massage all over. Gently pull ears in all directions. Squeeze the earlobe.

◆ Move hands back onto scalp. With frisky circular motion, massage scalp (as if you were shampooing the hair). Gently pull hair and then place hands over the scalp and hold for the count of ten.

For self-massage, *follow above instructions as you like. Remember: Combined with a head self-massage, this makes a great lead-in to a facial.*

Step Seven: Upper Chest, Arms and Hands

◆ Place 1 tablespoon of oil in palms of your hands and rub together to warm.

◆ Standing alongside the person, extend her arm and gently hold it at the wrist. With your other hand start from the wrist and glide up to the shoulder using a steady even pressure. Glide back down.

Repeat three times.

◆ Bend the person's arm so that it is resting across her tummy, palm down.

◆ Starting at the shoulder, knead the deltoids using the thumb and fingers from both hands. The thumbs should be at the center of the arm. Repeat twice.

◆ Move to the inside of the arm and repeat kneading motion on biceps.

◆ Next, place the palms of the hands on the top of the shoulder at the neck and smoothly and evenly rub outward to the top of the arm, then smooth over the bicep and down the elbow until you have a gentle hold on the hand.

◆ Ask the person to lift her left arm so that her fingers are pointing up at the ceiling.

◆ Rub the forearms from wrist to elbow using the thumbs.

◆ Take the wrist in your left hand.

Arm and Hand Self-Massage

If you are giving yourself a massage, do this last, to ease the accumulated stress.

- Start at the shoulder and move toward the fingertips using long, gliding strokes. Cover the inside and outside of the arm. Pay special attention to the area at the wrist—move through it firmly, pulling the tension through to the fingertips—pull the fingers out firmly and evenly—and then move the tension out of the body.

- Follow with a hand massage. Using two fingertips, rub the top and palm with rapid circular motions, going from the wrist toward the fingertips. Knead and pull the fingers. Repeat on other hand. Shake out fingers.

- Place your thumb on the palm of her hand and your fingers on the back of the hand. Move your thumbs in a firm circular motion.

- Gently grab each finger and pull it out from the hand. Rub and twist from the knuckle to the fingernail.

- Extend the arm down along the side of the person. Rub from wrist to shoulder in a long, firm stroke and glide back down. Repeat. Then feather down the arm using a tickling motion and clasp the hand in both of yours. Hold for the count of 10.

Repeat for other arm.

Step Eight: The Front of the Legs

+ Stand at the feet, facing up the body.
+ Repeat circulation and compression motions from Step Two.
+ Pour more oil in your hands. Starting at the ankle, place your hands so the fingers extend along the sides of the calf, thumbs along the top of the leg, fingertips along the outside. Smoothly, with long, gliding strokes, rub up the leg to the top of the thigh.

Repeat four times on each leg.

+ Working on the left leg, stand to the left side and place both of your hands, side by side, flat across the ankle.
+ Gently, but quickly, start rocking the leg back and forth with both hands.
+ Move your hands up the leg at a slow pace, rocking constantly. Be careful not to pull the skin.

Repeat on other leg. Rest. Repeat for both legs.

Note: You're now ready to do some deeper kneading of the muscles.

+ Standing by the left leg, slip your hands under the calf muscle. Grab the muscle firmly with your thumbs and fingers—they should be about 4 inches apart.

Squeeze fingers and thumb in toward each other slowly and with even pressure. As you do so, your well-oiled fingers and thumbs should ever so gently move across the muscle toward each other. If you hit a sore spot, you can hold at that point for the count of 5 and then move on.

Repeat that motion up the entire length of the calf and the thigh.

Repeat the long, gliding rub up the right leg.

Step Nine: The Feet

Foot massage can be approached as an extension of the techniques used in the full body massage or as a separate reflexology treatment. Reflexology correlates specific sections of the upper and lower foot with internal organs—and suggests that if you have a sensitivity in a certain part of your foot it may indicate some unsettledness in the corresponding organ. (However, just because your foot is tender to the touch in a specific spot does not mean that there is definitely something wrong in the corresponding organ.) Whichever type of foot rub you use, a foot massage can be a wonderfully relaxing and therapeutic interlude. And you can do it to yourself—or with a partner.

The Basic Massage

This foot massage will provide all-over relaxation.

* Have the person receiving the massage lie on her back with a pillow under the knees and the feet.
* Place lotion in hands and rub together, then apply thin coat of lotion to feet—tops and bottoms.
* Sitting comfortably facing the bottoms of the feet, grasp each foot in one of your hands, with your thumb on the arch and fingertips on the top of the foot. Gently massage and stimulate the feet, shaking them from side to side.
* Move hands to bottom of feet. Hook fingertips on top of ball of foot right under the bottom of the toes. Massage area gently with fingertips.
* Move hands to heels. Hold around heel and ankle, so you have a firm grip. Gently pull legs away from hip socket and shake from side to side.
* Place feet gently back on table.
* Place thumb in the center of the foot, directly below

the ball. Move thumbs in a circular motion pressing *through*, not down.

♦ You are now going to rub one foot at a time. Take the left foot in your hands. Place thumbs between the thin bones that extend from the toes up the foot. Rub in these spaces using long, steady pressure with the thumbs. First press from toes toward ankles, then reverse.

♦ Next, using both thumbs on the top of the foot, rub up the channels between the foot bones using a circular motion. Rub from the toes toward the ankle. Vibrate the foot as you rub.

♦ To finish up this phase of the massage, pull the foot gently but firmly out from leg and hip and bounce—gently. Rotate foot around ankle. Place on massage table.

Repeat for right foot.

♦ The toe rub comes next. Holding the foot in one hand, grasp the toes and rotate them gently from side to side. Then grab each toe separately and pull out from foot, then rotate.

♦ Move hand to arch of left foot. Resting the ball of your hand in the middle of the arch, thread your fingers through the toes. Wiggle from side to side. Then slowly and easily press toes and foot away from you to stretch the Achilles tendon.

Repeat for right foot.

♦ Finally, holding the left foot with left hand, place your right fist in arch of right foot. Starting below the toes, knead fist into arch all the way to the heel. Then, using the knuckle of the index finger, massage down a center line extending from between the second and third toes to the heel. Then slap bottom of foot with back of hand. Pull toes and gently stretch out foot. Let rest.

Repeat for the left foot.

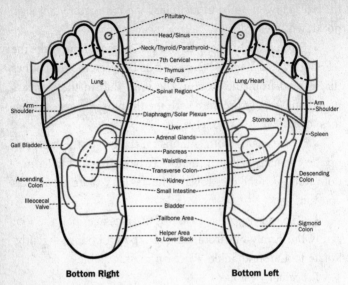

Illustration by Robin Michals.

Foot Reflexology

If you are interested in concentrating on a foot massage, try this wonderful, therapeutic technique that works on the whole body without ever having you leave the foot.

♦ Begin by relaxing both feet together using a combination of rubbing and pulling. (As on pages 122–23.)

♦ If you are having problems with your sinuses, or digestion, for example, find the corresponding location on the reflexology chart above and on the next page.

♦ Proceed using the four techniques described below:

Thumb walking: Using the outer edge of the thumbs, begin "walking" on the designated area. You may walk up and down on any part of the bottom of the foot from the base of the toes to the heel, and also from side to side on the heel and ball of foot. The technique also works on the ankle and upper foot areas. Press firmly and evenly, *through and out*—not down.

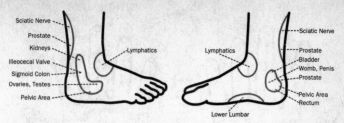

Illustration by Robin Michals.

Flat thumb circular rub: Place the fleshy parts of your thumbs over the area. Move thumbs in unison, pressing *through and out*, not down, as they circle the area.

The long stroke: Using your thumbs, press long and slowly across the area.

Rotate and pull: When you are finished rubbing the designated area, you should rotate and pull the toes and the whole foot, from the ankle.

Hand Reflexology

Hand reflexology correlates specific parts of the hands with internal organs. The chart on the next page will help direct you toward these areas. You can easily give yourself a hand massage—a great reward at the end of a long day at a keyboard. Use the same techniques as for the foot rub and foot reflexology massages outlined above. In addition:

♦   For a general hand massage, you may hold the hand in place by placing your fingers on the back of the hand, your thumb in center of the palm.

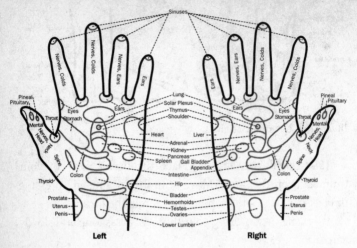

Illustration by Robin Michals.

♦ Apply a steady, even pressure downward with the padded part of the thumb. Once you have found the appropriate pressure, gently move the thumb in a circular motion all around the palm. Then move to each knuckle joint, massaging with finger below and thumb on top.

♦ If you are giving a hand massage to another person, use both thumbs, side by side. Move them over the area in opposite directions—the left thumb moving in a circle to the left, the right to the right.

Seven

·

Guided Meditation: For Body and Soul

Meditation is the practice of releasing and clearing the mind through relaxed concentration. Polished and perfected by the cultures of the Indian subcontinent, China and Japan, the art of meditation has now been recognized by Western medicine as an essential component of total health and well-being: Sitting in quiet, detached contemplation for twenty minutes a day can produce a profound effect on the cardiovascular system, management of pain and stress, and on mood and spirit.

Fortunately, you don't have to head for the mountaintop to enjoy these important benefits. Meditation can be integrated easily into your daily routine. You can meditate while you are walking to work, during a five-minute respite, or immediately before you fall asleep.

Meditation Basics

To help you get started, this chapter presents three *guided* meditations. We suggest that you record them for playback whenever you want to take a break. You can also have your spa partner read the routines to you. Either way, your goal is to make meditation a part of your daily schedule so that if you have insomnia, are angry or stressed out, feel creeping depression, or simply want to unwind after a long, hard day, you will have mastered this simple yet effective remedy.

Tips on Reading the Meditations Aloud

◆ Go slowly. Pause for many seconds between instructions, giving the mind and body time to fully respond to the images.

◆ Keep your voice soft and even, with minimal expression.

◆ When reciting or recording the meditations, you may want to play some music very softly in the background. Classical music is generally too stimulating and music with words can be highly distracting. Simple instrument solos or New Age music is your best choice.

◆ The guided meditations in this chapter are adapted from recorded meditations by Margaret Doner, L.M.T. If you'd like to order a prerecorded cassette, see the resource section on page 230.

Getting Started

♦   Sit, lie, or stand quietly for a couple of minutes before you begin. Allow your breath to become even and regular.

Begin by tuning into how you are breathing. Feel the air come in through your nostrils in long, slow, deep streams, filling up your lower lungs first, causing your belly to expand outward, then filling up the top of your lungs.

Feel the breath leave your lungs from the bottom upward, contracting your belly muscles gently as the air runs out. Let it escape through your slightly opened lips in an even stream.

You should exhale for almost twice as long as you inhale. For example, as you are breathing in try counting to 5, slowly and evenly. As you exhale, count to 10. This may be difficult to do at first. Don't force it. Start with an inhale of 3 to 4 and an exhale of 5 to 7. After practicing for a few days or a week, you may be able to increase your breaths without any effort.

♦   Let your focus on the world around you fade.

You may open or close your eyes—but you'll find it's particularly relaxing to close your eyes about ¾ of the way and allow the world to become fuzzy. Don't focus on anything in particular. Feel like a child whose eyelids have gotten very heavy, but who hasn't yet drifted off into sleep.

Meditation Routines

Once you have settled peacefully into a comfortable position and are breathing rhythmically and feel tranquil, you are ready to begin a guided meditation. The selection here includes a five-minute meditation to use whenever you need quick stress relief or rejuvenation; a seated fifteen-minute color meditation to lead you into deeper relaxation; a reclining meditation that can be used for the deepest relaxation and before going to sleep (it will overcome insomnia); and a walking meditation to demonstrate how easily meditation can be integrated into your everyday life.

Five-Minute Relaxer

◆

When you don't have time to do a long meditation, you can still gain many of the benefits—including stress reduction, increased cardiovascular health, and a boost to the immune system. The key is to lower your heart rate, deepen and slow your breathing, and clear your mind for five minutes. And if you're angry or frustrated, you'll find this brief meditation will keep you from saying or doing something you'll regret later.

Step One

◆ Sitting comfortably on a firm chair with a padded seat, plant your feet firmly on the ground. Feel your backbone, straight and well balanced, and your shoulders relaxed but not slumped forward. Your head is balanced perfectly.

◆ Take a deep breath, filling your lungs from the bottom, expanding them as they inflate. Now slowly and evenly expel the air, emptying the lungs from the bottom first, forcing the air up and out, feeling the lungs deflate and contract. Find a steady, even breath that you can sustain during the meditation.

Step Two

◆ Imagine that you can travel downward into the earth below your feet and begin to draw energy upward from the earth into the soles of your feet.

(Pause for the count of four.)

◆ Allow the energy to enter your body through your

feet. Feel it continue to move upward—past your ankles, into your legs.

(Pause for the count of four.)

♦ Let the energy rise up and wash through you—from your ankles to your knees. Fill your legs with grounding energy from the earth.

(Pause for the count of four.)

Step Three

♦ Continue to move the energy upward into your hips and torso. Feel it move freely up through the body, calming you, making you feel more grounded.

(Pause for the count of four.)

Step Four

♦ The energy is moving ever upward. Feel it reach your shoulders and neck. Feel how much tension is stored there. Let the energy dispel it.

♦ As the earth energy passes through the neck and shoulders, it lifts the tension off them and draws the tension upward through the head and out the top of the head.

♦ Send the tension on its way. Feel the energy stream move out of your body, upward to the sky.

(Pause for as long as you wish.)

Step Five

♦ Now that your body and mind are clear, fill them with the white pure energy of the sky. Bring it down from above and allow it to wash over the body. Feel the body glowing with beautiful white light. Surround yourself with this white light. The light pours into the earth.

(Pause for as long as you wish.)

♦ Feel your body washed clean by the earth and the

sky. All stress and anger wash away. You are ready to continue with your day.

Fifteen-Minute Seated Color Meditation

◆

This meditation is designed to be used as a regular part of your daily exercise and fitness routine, either after you do aerobics or whenever you find 15 minutes for yourself. In the spa programs in Chapter 10, this is the basic meditation that is recommended for use before receiving a massage, while having a facial, or to close the day's activities.

Step One

◆ Sit comfortably on a chair or the floor, with your back supported.

◆ Imagine a shimmering beam of white light coming down from above.

(Pause for the count of 5.)

◆ Feel the light enter the top of your head and watch it travel down your spine into the floor.

(Pause for 30 seconds.)

◆ Feel the light wash through your spine, clearing and cleaning it. Imagine the white light connecting you to the sky above and the ground below.

(Pause for 30 seconds.)

◆ Pull the light from the highest point in the sky and send it down into the earth to connect you to both the earth and the sky.

(Pause 30 seconds.)

Step Two

♦   Beginning in the lowest part of your abdomen, imagine a deep red light glowing. Fill the abdomen with a beautiful red light, imagining the light of a sunset, glowing deep within the body.

(Pause for at least 30 seconds—you may pause for several minutes if that suits you.)

♦   Begin to draw the light upward toward the navel. Just as the sunset turns from red to orange, the light in the abdomen turns from red to orange as it rises. The light glows deep orange and fills the upper abdomen.

(Pause for 30 seconds.)

Step Three

♦   The color continues to rise in the body. It becomes yellow at the solar plexus. Yellow like the sun.

(Pause for the count of 5.)

♦   It glows outward from the center of the body with a warm, yellow light.

(Pause for the count of 5.)

♦   Feel the warmth of the yellow light penetrating the middle of your body.

Step Four

♦   Bring the light up toward the heart. In the heart center it glows with a beautiful green color.

(Pause for at least 30 seconds.)

♦   Picture an emerald glowing in the center of your chest. This green color is expansive. It fills every corner of your chest.

(Pause for 30 seconds.)

Step Five

As the color rises to the throat, it becomes blue. Blue like the sky. It fills the throat and opens it. See the blue sky fill your throat.

(Pause for at least 30 seconds.)

Imagine the blue of the summer sky.

(Pause for at least 30 seconds.)

Step Six

The light rises up to the forehead, turning purple. A deep purple light radiates on the forehead, between the eyebrows, at the third eye.

(Pause for 5 seconds.)

Fill the forehead with a beautiful purple light. It glows like an amethyst.

(Pause for at least 10 seconds.)

Step Seven

♦ As the light continues upward to the crown of your head, it turns white again. It radiates up toward the sky from the top of your head.

(Pause for the count of 5.)

♦ Once you see the white light above your head in the sky, imagine pulling that light back down into your body.

(Pause for the count of 5.)

♦ Imagine that the body acts as a prism, breaking the light into colors: purple, blue, green, yellow, orange, and red. It travels back down through your body into the earth. Your body is a rainbow of living colors. Feel it glowing.

(Pause for 30 seconds.)

♦ You are at peace and completely relaxed. Held between earth and sky in perfect contentment.

(Pause for the count of 5.)

Step Eight

♦   Reflect upon your day. Are you holding anger or resentment? Take a deep breath and release your anger. Release the resentment. Release the stress. Send it on its way.

(Pause for 90 seconds.)

♦   Reflect on your body. Are you holding tension anywhere? Take a deep breath and release the tension. Let it go, send it on its way.

(Pause for 90 seconds.)

♦   Repeat after me: "I am calm and relaxed. My mind is clear."

(Pause for the count of 5.)

♦   "My body is clear."

(Pause for the count of 5.)

♦   "I am at peace." Repeat these words to yourself, silently. Continue to repeat as long as you feel you want to.

♦   You are now calm and relaxed and ready to rejoin the world. You may open your eyes.

Journey of the Peaceful Rest

♦

This guided meditation is guaranteed to send you off to dreamland and banish the tension from your body and your face. In a half- or full-day spa routine, this meditation is an essential part of the experience.

Step One

♦   Make sure you are resting comfortably on your back with a pillow under your knees to ease lower back strain.

Breathe deeply through your nose and exhale through your mouth. Feel your lower torso inflate with air as you inhale and fall as you exhale. With each exhale, feel your day's tensions drift away.

(Pause for 30 seconds.)

Step Two

♦ Imagine a warm sunlight coming down from above. Golden, warm light beaming down from above. It touches the top of your head and relaxes away the tension in your scalp.

(Pause for 30 seconds.)

♦ Feel the sunlight melt away the tension.

♦ The warm glow moves down into the temples and forehead, warming and relaxing them.

(Pause.)

♦ The golden light melts the tension away and it runs off your body, draining away into the earth below you.

(Pause for as long as feels comfortable.)

♦ Continue to imagine the light bathing your face. The cheeks, jaw, mouth, and chin relax completely as they are bathed by the warm glow of the sun.

(Pause.)

♦ Feel your entire face and head warmed and relaxed by the sun.

(Pause for 60 seconds.)

Step Three

♦ As the golden, warm sunlight moves down the body, it fills the neck and throat with its soothing presence. Feel the warm sun; feel it melt tension away from the body. Feel the neck and throat relax and open.

(Pause 30 seconds.)

♦ Continue to imagine the light traveling ever so slowly down the length of the body. As it touches the chest and shoulders, feel them relax and release. Let the tension melt away. The golden light fills the chest and shoulders inside and out and relaxes them.

(Pause 30 seconds.)

Step Four

♦ Now the sun fills the center of your body. The stomach is relaxed and warm. The golden light glows onto the body and warms it.

(Pause.)

♦ The stomach relaxes as the sun spreads into the hips.

(Pause.)

♦ Your body is relaxed and at rest. Imagine a beautiful spring day. The sun penetrates and relaxes your body and mind.

(Pause 30 seconds.)

Step Five

♦ The hips and thighs are now warmed by the sun. The legs feel its penetrating warmth. They relax. The tension slides off.

(Pause.)

♦ The whole body glows with sunlight; you feel warmed and relaxed.

(Pause 60 seconds.)

Step Six

♦ As your body relaxes and releases the tension it becomes lighter and lighter. All resistance is removed. All the tension is removed. As the body becomes lighter, it begins to float. It lifts off the earth, like a cloud, and floats upward into the sky.

(Pause for at least 1 minute.)

♦ Like a cloud your body drifts easily through the sky.

The sun warms it. The wind shifts it easily. All resistance is removed.

(Pause for at least 30 seconds.)

♦   Your body, now a cloud, travels easily through the sky.

(Pause for at least 1 minute.)

♦   You float over the earth like a bird. Freely you float, easy and relaxed. Warmed by the sun, moved by the gentle breeze.

(Pause for at least 30 seconds.)

♦   A gentle bird passes by, singing sweetly. Below you, a stream bubbles along. The green earth greets the sunlight. Your body travels and drifts above it. You are at peace.

(Pause.)

♦   You travel to a beautiful land. In this land is relaxation and rest. Everything flows smoothly in the land. Spend some time in the land of peace and quiet. Spend some time in the land of rest and happiness. Relax. Be still.

(Pause for about 2 minutes.)

♦   You may end your journey by awakening or continuing on to sleep. If you choose to awaken, do so by counting slowly to 5 and opening your eyes at the count of 5. If you choose to sleep, continue your journey into the land of peaceful rest.

Walking Meditation

♦

Walking at a smooth pace, with an even, measured gait, can become meditative, especially when you join it with deep, peaceful breathing and focused thoughts. Choose a location for your stroll that is free of traffic and difficult terrain.

Step One

♦ Begin walking purposefully but in a slow, smooth rhythm. Don't rush; don't dawdle.

♦ Step solidly, but without hitting the ground. Let your arms move naturally at your sides, swinging freely. Walk with your shoulders relaxed, not hunched up to the ears. Keep your torso erect and stomach muscles tight enough to hold you upright comfortably. Breathe and stroll—nice and easy—in and out, as you stride, gliding forward.

Step Two

♦ Focus your eyes on the landscape around you. Instead of passing by without noticing, pay attention to the individual leaves on the trees, the texture of the grass, the configurations of the clouds and the quality of the light.

(Pause in reading for 60 seconds.)

Step Three

♦ Keep striding comfortably. Feel the air against your skin. Is it warm or cool? Damp or dry? Is there a wind? Does it offer resistance or is it at your back? Feel the air around you and feel it passing in and out of your lungs, making you part of the scene.

(Pause in reading for 30 seconds.)

Step Four

♦ Turn your attention to your body. Beginning with your feet, tune into how they are feeling. Are they tired? Cramped? Happy to be walking?

(Pause in reading for 10 seconds.)

♦ Move your focus up both your legs, feeling your calves and thighs, your pelvic region, your torso. Sense areas of tension, feel the muscles working. Take deep breaths and exhale slowly, expelling the tension. Put a spring in your step. Make your walk more lively.

(Pause in reading for 1 minute.)

◆ Now think about your back. Your stomach muscles support your back and take the strain and pressure off it. Lift your abdominals and use them to support your body. Feel your body straighten and become taller as you walk. But keep your shoulders relaxed and low.

(Pause briefly in reading.)

Step Five

◆ Swing your arms easily by your sides. Focus on the easy, loose motion. Now make your hands rigid, fingers tensed until they quiver. Then let your fingers go limp and shake your hands from the wrist, letting your fingers flop.

(Pause briefly in reading.)

Step Six

◆ Tune into your breathing again. As you exhale, feel the tension in your body dissipate from your legs, your torso, your shoulders and arms.

(Pause in reading for 10 seconds.)

Step Seven

◆ Now relax your neck and head. Let your head fall forward, chin toward chest. Gently swing it from left to right, shoulder to shoulder.

◆ Turn your head slowly so you are looking over your right and then left shoulder.

(Pause in reading for the count of 5.)

◆ Tip your head right to left, trying to touch your ears to your shoulders.

(Pause in reading for the count of 5.)

♦ Lift your hands up and scratch your scalp vigorously. Rub your head and face. Let all the tension go.

(Pause in reading for the count of 5.)

♦ Return your focus to the world around you. Notice the details of your surroundings. Walk through the world aware of its glory. Rejoin the world around you.

Eight

Body Workout: Stretching, Toning, and Conditioning Routines

Exercise is meant to be a part of your everyday life: Tending the garden, walking the dog, chasing after the kids, playing tennis, enjoying yoga, jogging or swimming—all qualify as exercise. Each such activity helps you embrace the pleasure of using your body and keeps it toned and supple. But many of us work long hours at a desk and collapse in the evening in front of the TV. In fact, over 70 percent of us are inactive or exercise only sporadically. But we can make enormous improvements in our well-being with minimal effort. Just thirty minutes a day—and it doesn't have to be all at once—of physical activity, such as vacuuming, walking up stairs, or chasing the kids around, has a far-reaching impact on our health.

At The Wellness Center we try to encourage people to find the activities that work for them—and then stick with them. So, for your home spa experience, we've created a basic program that provides a taste of the pleasures of stretching, toning and aerobics. Theses forms of exercise work together to help you:

- Dispel stress
- Beautify your skin
- Tone your body
- Raise your spirits

If you are not already a dedicated exerciser, perhaps doing these simple and enjoyable routines will help you make room for exercise in your life.

Body Toning Exercises
designed by Margaret Doner

Stretching, toning, and aerobics are an important part of any spa experience. *Stretching* frees your energy and helps prevent exercise-related injuries to muscles, tendons and ligaments. Stretching should come both before and after the toning and aerobics portions of a workout.

Toning comes from doing repetitions of light, weight-bearing exercises. It gives you strength and endurance as well as shapely muscles and smooth, healthy skin.

Aerobics are essential for cardiovascular health. They help reduce stress, regulate hormone levels, and move your energy so it can nurture all parts of your mind, body and spirit.

However, excess exercise of any kind produces stress, depletes the body, and can damage joints and muscles and tendons. Regular, moderate activity is the key to long-term good health.

FYI

Q. Do I need to call my doctor before I start an exercise program?
A. You must see a doctor if you're over 40, over 35 and on the Pill or have never exercised, if you smoke, are overweight, or have heart trouble, chest pain, high blood pressure, or any serious medical condition.

Q. I hate to exercise. I hate to even move! Is there any hope for me?
A. Of course! The newest research demonstrates that if you are basically fit, all you need to stay healthy is about 30 minutes of exercise three days a week—and you don't have to do it all at once. According to the Centers for Disease Control and Prevention and the American College of Sports Medicine, these 30 minutes don't have to be consecutive: 10 minutes of gardening, a 15-minute walk, and five minutes up and down the stairs will improve your general health and lower your risk of life-threatening illnesses, especially if you now do nothing at all.

However, the more vigorously you work out, the better the results will be. And it will take some effort. There's no genie who will exercise for you! Probably the most

Tip: If you are enjoying an at-home spa with a friend, you may want to read the exercise routines aloud to each other. Or you can tape record them for playback when you want to work out.

important thing you can do is to make exercise a habit, like brushing your teeth. It's easier to do when it's part of your regular routine. Start slowly for best results. You'll be less likely to burn out if you don't use up all your enthusiasm right away, plus it's better for your body to get in shape gradually.

Q. I play on my company softball team and I'm not over-weight. Does that mean I'm fit?
A. You can be slim and still be out of shape. And softball and bowling, two of Americas' most popular sports, don't contribute to aerobic fitness. A simple test: Run in place for 30 seconds then take your pulse. If it's above your target heart rate (see box, page 154), you need to exercise regularly.

Q. Should I join a health club?
A. The advantages: one-on-one help; more equipment and facilities than a home gym; options such as massages and whirlpools. The disadvantages: it's the most expensive exercise choice; you can only go when it's open, which may be inconvenient; you may feel self-conscious, which can mean you'll drop out. What you decide to do depends on what will work for you.

#1 Stretching

Getting Comfortable
- Start in a neutral standing position. Feel your shoulders relax and your abdominals tighten, supporting your lower and upper back. Breathe deeply through your nose and exhale through your mouth. Feel the diaphragm expand when

you inhale and contract when you exhale. Don't lift the shoulders. Repeat until your breath comes without stress.

The Big Body Bend

♦   As you inhale, raise your arms to the ceiling, fingers pointing upward, palms facing each other.

♦   On the exhale, lower your arms in front of your body. Feel the weight of your arms pulling your shoulders forward, rounding them slightly and making your chin lower to your chest, your head bend forward slightly, and your eyes look to your toes.

♦   Then gently bend at the waist, extending your hands downward so that they are dangling about shin high, 6 inches from the floor. Keep breathing.

♦   On an inhale, slowly raise your back, keeping your shoulders rounded and head bent forward until you are almost in an upright position. As you become erect, lift the head. At the same time, extend the arms above the head. Repeat the entire motion.

Side Stretch

♦   Stand with your feet about 10 inches apart, toes forward, arms at your sides.

♦   Extend your left hand and arm up to the ceiling. At the same time, bend to your right so that your right arm and fingers point toward the floor.

♦   Curving the left hand over your head so that your fingers are pointing toward the right wall and the left side of your torso is stretched fully, hold for the count of ten— breathing in and out all the while.

♦   Slowly stand upright, bringing your left arm back down along your left side.

♦   Repeat for the other side.

Waist Stretch

+ Standing comfortably with feet parallel, about 10 inches apart, bend arms and place hands at waist.
+ Breathing out, bend forward about 45 degrees and then rotate your torso so that you trace a circle, moving from the front, to the right side, straight up, and to the left side.
+ Reverse direction of the circle.
+ Repeat 2 times.

Shoulder and Arm Rotation

+ Moving your arms in unison, slowly rotate them forward in a windmill motion from top to front to bottom and then back.
+ Repeat 3 times.
+ Reverse direction, repeat 3 times.
+ Let arms hang down at sides. Shake fingers.

Neck Noodle

+ Standing comfortably and breathing evenly, tilt the head so the left ear is moving toward the left shoulder. Hold for count of 4.
+ Pick up head and move it smoothly from side to side so that the right ear is moving toward the right shoulder. Hold for count of 4.
+ Repeat the pair 3 times.

Calf Flex and Achilles Tendon Warm-Up

+ Stand on a step and let heels drop down below the step. Hold onto hand railing. (A thick book will do, too.)
+ Then stand securely on your left foot and pick your right foot off the floor.
+ Now rotate the right foot at the ankle in a full circle several times to loosen the joints and tendons.
+ Repeat on left foot.

#2 Toning

Upper Body Muscle Work
♦ You can use soup cans if you don't have hand weights available. Recommended weights: 2, 3, or 5 pounds in each hand. It's repetition of motion that tones the muscles, not hefting weight.

Biceps Pumping
♦ Stand comfortably with feet parallel, shoulders relaxed but not droopy or sagging forward. Your knees should be slightly bent.

♦ Grip a weight in each hand, arms extended straight down along the sides of your body.

♦ Slowly bring the weights up to your chest, bending at the elbow with palms facing upward. Exhale as you bring them up. Then slowly lower them, inhaling. Remember to keep your stomach and abdominal muscles tight—you want to use your stomach muscles, not your back muscles, to hold you upright and relaxed. Repeat 10 times. Rest for count of 10. Repeat 10 more times.

♦ To speed up the tempo, repeat exercise with one arm at a time, alternating rapidly, one after the other. Repeat 10 times. Rest for count of 10. Repeat 10 more times.

Put down weights. Shake out arms and hands. Shrug your shoulders. Pick up weights again.

Deltoids
♦ Standing comfortably with your arms at your sides, holding the weights, extend your arms straight out from your sides until your arms are parallel with the floor, and your palms—grasping the weights—are facing down toward the floor. Keep arms slightly below shoulder level.

- Lower arms halfway. Hold for count of 3. Lower the rest of the way. Repeat series 10 times.
- Now extend arms up to shoulder level and lower so they are straight at your sides in one slow, smooth motion. Repeat 10 times.

For Toning Flabby Underarms

- Holding the weights, draw both arms behind your back, keeping the upper arm in contact with the body and the wrists facing in toward each other.
- Keeping the upper arm lifted behind the body and tightly pressed to your side, bend the elbow and bring the weight up to your shoulder. Hold for count of two and return to original position and hold for count of two. You may do both arms at the same time. Repeat 10 times, rest, and repeat another 10. Rest.
- Assume your beginning position with both arms extended out behind you, wrists parallel. Pulse both arms up and down for a count of 10, rest, and repeat series twice.

The Big Circle

- Lie down on the floor, on your back. Bend knees and plant feet firmly on the floor. Keep your abdominal muscles tight and extend your arms out to the side so they are resting on the floor straight out from your shoulders. Lift both arms (including the upper arm) slightly off the floor.
- Slowly bring your slightly bowed arms up so your fingertips meet above your chest and your arms are creating a big circle.

Lower arms to the floor. Repeat 10 times.

- Pick arms off floor about 6 inches. Hold to side and pulse up and down for the count of 10. Repeat 10 times. Lower arms. Rest. Repeat the entire exercise.

Lower Body Muscle Work

You may want to use strap-on ankle weights to increase the workout.

Seated Leg Lift

◆ Sit on the floor with your legs extended straight out in front of you.

◆ Bend your left knee until your thigh is parallel to your chest. Grab that leg with your arms and hold on firmly. Leave your right leg extended out straight in front of you.

◆ Raise the right leg straight up from the floor with the toe pointing to the ceiling. If you can only get it up an inch, that's fine—whatever you can do will work the muscles for you. Repeat 10 times, raising and then returning to the floor. Then raise the leg and hold it for the count of 3. Pulse it without touching the floor 10 times. Rest.

◆ Repeat the exercise with the other leg.

◆ Repeat entire exercise again.

Side Leg Lift

◆ Lie on the floor along your left side. Cradle your head on your left arm. Bend your left leg so it forms a triangle with your right leg to brace and stabilize you. Place your right hand on the floor in front of you to help keep you steady.

◆ Lift up the right leg as high as you can with the knee facing front. Keep the leg straight and the foot flexed. Repeat 10 times. Rest. Repeat 10 more times.

◆ Now rotate the leg so the knee, instead of facing forward, is facing more toward the ceiling. Lift the straight leg as high as you can 10 times. Rest. Repeat.

Inside Thigh Tightener

◆ Lying on the floor along your left side, bend your right knee and plant your right foot firmly on the floor in front of your left leg. (Some of you will place it near the mid-shin, others up by the knee or thigh. Do what's comfortable.)

♦   Prop your head up by putting your left elbow on the floor and resting your left ear in the palm of your left hand. When you feel steady and comfortable . . .

♦   Raise your left leg up off the floor, keeping your foot flexed and your knee softly straightened (don't overextend the knee). Repeat this upward motion 10 times. Rest. Repeat.

♦   Raise your left leg up off the floor and pulse it 10 times. Rest and repeat.

♦   Repeat the exercise on the other side. Increase the number of leg raises to find the point at which you are seriously taxing the muscle.

Bottom Squeeze

♦   Lie on your back and bend both knees so that your feet are planted firmly on the floor as close to your bottom as is comfortable.

♦   Lift your rear end off the floor and form a bridge by resting on your shoulder blades. Pulse the pelvis toward the ceiling. Repeat 10 times. Rest. Repeat exercise twice more.

Stomach Firming Exercises

Toning the stomach muscles is difficult—sometimes it seems like you need super stomach muscles just to do the strengthening exercises. There are many products on the market you can buy to make the workout easier and more effective. But you can get just as good results with the old-fashioned routines given below.

Crunch

The crunch is a great exercise—in fact nothing tightens the abs as well. But it can also cause a lot of back trouble if you do it wrong.

Rule #1: Don't do a "full sit-up." Never come all the way up to a sitting position.

Rule #2: Don't do crunches with your legs out straight. Always have knees bent and feet flat on the floor.

+ Lie down on the floor with the knees bent. Inhale. Place your hands on your abdominal area.

As you exhale, press your stomach into the floor and tighten your abdominal muscles. Feel the tightening with your hands. Hold for count of 5. Inhale. Exhale. Rest. Repeat.

+ Inhale. Place your hands behind your head with elbows extended to the side, and with knees bent. Raise the shoulders and upper torso off the floor by pressing the stomach muscles into the floor and exhaling. Repeat 10 times. Rest. Repeat 10 times. Rest.

The lift of the body should come from contraction of stomach muscles, not through strain on your back, shoulder, and neck.

+ Next, with hands behind your head and elbows out to the side, lift the body and twist so that your left elbow extends toward the right knee. Lie back down. Remember to exhale as you bend and twist; inhale as you lie down.

Repeat with other elbow and knee.

Repeat both sides 10 times. Rest. Repeat entire exercise.

#3 Aerobics

It doesn't matter how you get your aerobic exercise—what matters is that you do get it regularly for between 25 and 45 minutes.

+ If you prefer to get your aerobic workout in a class situation, you can follow the program that's laid out for you in this section.

• If you have an exercise bicycle, treadmill, or cross-country ski machine at home, enjoy a 25–45-minute workout as part of your comprehensive spa treatment.

• You also can head outdoors for a brisk 25–45-minute walk, jog, skate, or other outdoor sport. The chart below shows that you don't need expensive equipment or a pricey gym to reap the health benefits of cardiovascular exercises. Simply walking can protect your health.

Miles Walked Per Week

	5–10	10–16	16–21	21–26	26–31	31–36	OVER 36
Decrease in risk of death	22%	27%	37%	38%	48%	54%	38%

♦ Based on a study of 17,000 Harvard alumni

However you choose to exercise, the object of aerobic activity is to raise your heart rate so that you increase your respiration, exercise the heart muscle, and increase your stamina. But you can overdo it—which strains the heart and makes the body less efficient at burning calories and fat. So whenever you do aerobics, if you're basically fit, you should aim for the target heart rates given in the chart on page 154.

Listen to the Music
• Put on your favorite up-tempo music—it can be anything from rap to swing.

• Start out marching in place. Raise your knees as high as you can with each step. You should be stepping at as fast a rate as you can sustain for 5 minutes.

• After 5 minutes shift into a skip. Repeat for 5 minutes.

• Now march in place for 30 steps.

• Keep marching but begin swinging your arms

Determine Your Target Heart Rate

To improve your stamina and performance, your pulse while doing aerobic exercise should range from 60% to 80% of your maximum heart rate, which is determined by subtracting your age from 220.

AGE	MAXIMUM HEART RATE	TARGET HEART RATE ZONE	
		60%	80%
25	195	117	156
30	190	114	152
35	185	111	148
40	180	108	144
45	175	105	140
50	170	102	136
55	165	99	132
60	160	96	128
65	155	93	124
70	150	90	120

• Check your pulse about 10 minutes into your workout or take the talk test—if you're too breathless to speak, you're working too hard. You shouldn't be able to sing or whistle.

• Check your pulse on your wrist, with your finger not your thumb. Count pulses for 15 seconds (the first beat is 0 not 1) then multiply by 4.

from front to back, describing a half circle. Continue for 30 more steps.

• Now slide sideways one long step and close your feet together. Repeat to the other side. Get in a rhythm and repeat back and forth, side to side, for 20 times on each side.

- Do 25 jumping jacks.
- March in place for 30 steps or longer, until your breathing is slowed down.
- Head for the stairs. If you're in a two-story house, use the inside stairs. In an apartment building take advantage of the building stairs. Begin slowly, taking care not to jar your knees. Walk up the stairs until it is uncomfortable or you are winded. Pause. Walk down the same distances. Pause.
- Repeat as many times as you can without overtaxing your cardiovascular system or your knees. (If you have heart disease or chronic knee trouble, skip this exercise.) Your goal is 10 minutes of walking up and down without pausing—but you may want to work up to that slowly. If no stairs are available, repeat the skipping routine from above.

#4 Advanced Stretching/Après Workout

When you do these stretches, do *not* bounce, and remember to breathe smoothly—exhaling on the stretch.

Leg Ease
- Sitting on the floor, place the soles of your feet together with the knees bent and as close to the floor as you can comfortably get them. Hold onto your ankles with your hands. You can rest your forearms along your calves.
- Round your shoulders and drop your chin to your chest.

Calorie Burning

These numbers are for a 130-pound woman. You'll burn 5% more calories for every 7 pounds over 130 that you weigh; 5% fewer calories for every 7 pounds under 130.

ACTIVITY	CALORIES BURNED PER 1/2 HOUR
Aerobic dancing	210
Cycling 8 miles	150
Gardening	150
Housecleaning	126
Running 3 miles	300
Sitting	42
Sunbathing	36
Swimming	261
Tennis	222
Volleyball	102
Walking 2 miles	150

Lower the head toward the ankles. Slowly. Exhaling. Hold. Then release slowly.

♦   Repeat 3 times.

Front Stretch

♦   Still sitting on the floor, extend your legs out in front of you.

♦   Bend your left leg so that the bottom of your foot is resting against the inside of your right knee.

♦   Inhale.

♦   Stretching your arm out in front of you, bend over and reach for your right foot. Round your back. Keep your chin bent toward your chest. Repeat 5 times.

♦   Switch legs. Repeat.

Information Please!

For helpful literature on exercise and health call or write: American College of Sports Medicine (ACSM), P.O. Box 1440, Indianapolis, IN 46202; 317-637-9200 ext. 127. Their booklets include "Fitness in Healthy Adults" and "Weight-Loss Programs."

The President's Council on Physical Fitness and Sports, Washington D.C. 20001; 202-272-3421.

American Heart Association, 7320 Greenville Avenue, Dallas, TX.

Consumer Information Center Publications, U.S. General Services Administration, Washington D.C. 20405, 202-501-1794, publishes on a wide variety of fitness and health topics.

Wishbone

♦   Sit on the floor with your back straight and your legs opened up in as wide a V as you can hold comfortably. They should be straight, knees comfortable and touching the floor.

♦   Extend the right arm up into the air over your head and then slowly bend forward at an angle so that you reach toward—or maybe touch—your left ankle. Hold for the count of 4.

♦   Slowly circle your arm from your left ankle to the floor in front of you. Keep your torso rounded forward and bend your head as close to the floor as possible.

♦   Sit up slowly and repeat for the other arm and leg.

Clothespin

 •   Bring your legs together so you're sitting on the floor with your back straight. (You can hold yourself up with your hands behind you on the floor if you need.)

 •   Bend forward—bringing your arms forward, too.

 •   Stretch toward your toes, reaching with your hands to your ankles. Grab onto your knees, shins, or wherever you can reach. Remember, do not bounce. Stretch slowly, exhaling as you go further—holding your place as you inhale.

 •   When you are as far forward as is comfortably possible, hold for a count of 5.

 •   Release your hands slowly and curl back up to a sitting position. Repeat 5 times.

Back Ease

 •   Lie flat on your back and bring both knees to your chest.

 •   Curl your arms around your shins and hold on.

 •   Rest there, breathing evenly and regularly, for the count of at least 10. You may want to hold this for up to a minute if your back is sore or if the stretch feels particularly good.

Sidewinder

 •   Lying on the floor with your legs straight, bend your left knee and place the left foot on the outside of the right knee. Flop your left knee over your right leg, toward the floor.

 •   Keep your shoulders on the floor with arms relaxed but extended out from the body. Hold this for 30 seconds. Repeat to other side.

Nine

·

Spa Cuisine for Everyday Healthy Eating

Some of the country's leading spas offer exotic Pacific Rim cuisine, others serve vegetarian delights, and some prepare inventive, streamlined versions of traditional American cooking. But what unifies all the styles is that they reflect a commitment to low-fat, high-flavor, palate-pleasing dishes that make it irresistible to eat healthful foods. In fact, today, spa cuisine is in the culinary vanguard, teaching Americans how to select and prepare gourmet meals that please the eye and satisfy the taste buds without resorting to excess fat, meat protein, or empty calories.

At the finest spas, menu plans come with the spa package—and mealtimes are often part of the rituals of renewal.

These facilities practice what the ancient Chinese healers taught: that food must be eaten in a serene environment if it is to be properly digested and provide the body with the balanced energy it needs. Eating should never be simply something to do between body wraps.

Once you've become familiar with this innovative approach to food, you won't want to limit your enjoyment of it to those rare times you are visiting a facility or creating an at-home spa experience. Healthful, delicious foods should be the foundation of every meal, every day. To help you expand your culinary expertise, this chapter offers samples of easy-to-prepare beverages, snacks, cold entrées, main courses, and desserts. We also set out spa menus for breakfast, lunch, and dinner that you can follow during your at-home spa sessions. They are designed to give you a choice of calorie totals, depending on how much energy you are expending in a day. If you're lolling in a warm tub, enjoying a massage, facial, and pedicure, you can choose the lower calorie menus. For those of you who engage in vigorous aerobic exercise during your spa session, the higher calorie menus are designed to keep up your energy. We hope that whatever recipes you choose to make, they will serve as a guide, inspiring you to explore the wonderful flavors and tastes that are available in gourmet low-fat, high-nutrition foods.

The rewards of following a spa cuisine diet plan are far-reaching. You will enjoy better digestion, more energy, lower cholesterol levels, weight loss, healthier skin, and a more satisfying sex life. The dangers of ignoring the guidelines are as equally profound. The Surgeon General's Report on Nutrition and Health reveals that five of the top ten causes of death in America—coronary heart disease, some types of cancer, stroke, diabetes, and atherosclerosis—may be related to dietary habits. In addition, many women's diseases, such as breast and endometrial cancer, are linked to obesity. Diet also plays a role in osteoporosis, some forms of arthritis, and migraines. There's no area of your health that isn't affected by what you eat.

6 Steps to a Healthier Diet

1. Cut the fat.
2. Eat a wide variety of foods.
3. Increase consumption of vegetables, fruits, grains, and and beans.
4. Make meat, chicken, and fish a side dish, not the main course.
5. Whenever possible eat organic produce and chemical-free meats and chicken.
6. Drink at least 8 glasses of water a day.

What do these six rules mean in practice?

♦ In the morning, on your bagel have 1 tablespoon of raspberry jelly, not cream cheese, and save 50 calories and 10 grams of fat. That's 5 pounds a year that you can lose without much effort or sacrifice.

♦ For lunch, try a turkey sandwich on whole grain bread, topped with lettuce, tomato, and mustard, instead of mayo and Swiss cheese. You'll save 185 calories and 18 grams fat. Save that many calories every day for a year and you've eliminated 19 pounds' worth!

♦ For dinner, have broiled skinless chicken, steamed spinach, and a tossed salad with no-fat dressing in place of spaghetti and meatballs. You'll save 520 calories and 21 grams of fat. Do that every night, in addition to the changes at break-

Targeting a Healthy Amount of Fat in Your Daily Meals

	◆ 30% CALORIES FROM FAT	◆ 25% CALORIES FROM FAT	◆ 20% CALORIES FROM FAT
1,400 calories a day	46 fat grams	39 fat grams	31 fat grams
1,600 calories a day	53 fat grams	44 fat grams	35 fat grams
1,800 calories a day	60 fat grams	50 fat grams	40 fat grams
2,000 calories a day	66 fat grams	55 fat grams	44 fat grams

fast and lunch, and you'll not only hit any weight loss goal you have, you'll lower your cholesterol dramatically.

Tip: A healthy diet is not about starving, or eliminating entire categories of food from your meals. It's about moderation, variety, and a love of fine flavors.

Your Daily Goals

Sedentary women (and that's 70 percent of us) may eat around 1,600 calories a day—and no more than 480 calories (30 percent of your daily total) should come from fat. (One gram of fat equals 9 calories, so you want to eat between 35 and 53 grams of fat.) But whatever your level of activity, it's generally not a good idea to consume less than 1,200 to 1,400 calories a day—even on a weight-loss plan. Eating fewer than that will make it more difficult to take in sufficient nutrients and to create lean muscle and burn fat.

Active women can increase their calorie intake to around 2,200 calories—but should try to limit fat to no more than about 67 grams, or less than 30 percent of the total intake. The American Heart Association recommends that your fat consumption goal should be to limit fat to 30 percent of your daily calories. Many nutritionists suggest that 25 percent is even better. For those who are working to reduce cholesterol levels and lose weight, limiting fat intake to 20 percent of calories for the day should produce steady, dramatic results.

Unfortunately, most Americans take in between 37 and 40 percent of their daily calories from fat. In fact, the average sedentary adult takes in around 75 grams of fat a day—that's 141,255 excess fat calories a year!

Fat Facts

Fat is not all bad: Some types—polyunsaturated and mono-unsaturated—help the body clear heart-stopping lipoproteins and cholesterol from the bloodstream. But don't start thinking there's such a thing as a safe fat. They're all calorie-intense and can lead to obesity, which in turn leads to all sorts of life-threatening illnesses. Stick with the least harmful fats, but be moderate at all times.

Okay Oils

The oils with the most unsaturated fats are canola, almond, safflower, sunflower, corn, olive, walnut, and sesame. Safflower is highest in polyunsaturated fats. Olive oil is highest in monounsaturated, which are the most effective in removing harmful cholesterol from the bloodstream.

Saturated fat is bad because it keeps the body from clearing cholesterol out of the bloodstream. It is found in the greatest amounts in animal products, commercial baked goods, dairy foods, and cheese. Vegetable oils also contain some saturated fats.

Bad Oils

Coconut, palm kernel, butter, cocoa butter, palm, and cotton-seed are the vegetable oils with the most saturated fat. Coconut oil is a whopping 92 percent saturated fat! In contrast, canola is only 7 percent saturated fat.

The American Heart Association (AHA) recommends that less than 10 percent of your total daily calories come from saturated fats. (Aim for 7 percent for best health.) If you're eating 1,600 calories a day, that's the equivalent of a little more than two tablespoons of butter or a twelve-ounce T-bone (trimmed of fat). Remember: Almost half the fat in beef is saturated.

The AHA also recommends that you keep polyunsaturated fats to 10 percent or less of your daily calories. Polyunsaturated fats are found in vegetable oils and some fish, such as herring, anchovies, pink salmon, tuna, sardines, and mackerel, which are also high in heart-healthy Omega-3 fatty acids. Monounsaturated fats, which are found in the greatest quantities in olives, peanuts, and avocados, and the oils made from those plants, should make up the rest of the total fat intake—about 10 to 15 percent of total calories.

So What's Cholesterol?

Cholesterol is a waxy white substance that the body requires to manufacture sex hormones and build cells. All the choles-

Cholesterol Goals

	DESIRABLE	BORDERLINE	UNDESIRABLE
Total	below 200	200–239	240+
LDL	below 130	130–159	160+
HDL	above 45 (above 60 reduces risk of heart disease)	35–45	below 35

terol our body needs is produced by the liver. We take in extra cholesterol when we eat meats, dairy products, poultry, and fish. When we consume too much, a lot may stick to our artery walls. The possible result—a heart attack or stroke.

There are two types of cholesterol: LDL, which sticks to your arteries and hurts your heart, and HDL, which helps the body "unstick" the LDL and excrete it from the body. The newest research reveals that your HDL level is as important as your overall cholesterol level for predicting potential cardio-vascular problems.

A low overall cholesterol count with low HDLs is not healthy. You want to aim for low total cholesterol and high HDLs.

Tip: You should take in no more than 300 mg of cholesterol a day. And the National Cholesterol Education Program recommends that everyone be tested for overall cholesterol and HDL levels—once at age 20 and then every 5 years.

How to Lower Your Total Cholesterol and Raise Your HDLs

- Lose weight. Losing weight raises HDL levels.
- Eat more fiber—1 bowl of oatmeal a day may lower overall cholesterol 2 to 3 percent.
- One (and only one) drink of alcohol a day may raise HDL.
- Exercise. Vigorous exercise may raise HDL up to 20 percent.
- Quit smoking. Quitting smoking dramatically increases HDL levels.
- Reduce overall consumption of fats and increase amount of fat from monounsaturated oils such as olive oil.

Beware Hidden Fat

You may know that there is a lot of fat in red meat and fried foods. But fat is hidden in all kinds of foods:

Potato chips. Sixty percent of their calories are from fat. If you eat one ounce (about 16 chips)—and you know you can't eat just a handful—you'll take in 10 grams of fat. That's almost a quarter of a day's fat for many of us. Alternatives? Pretzels are just as crunchy, with almost no fat; low-fat chips are available, or oven-bake tortillas until they're crispy and season them with garlic powder, red pepper, or a very thin dusting of Parmesan cheese.

Salad dressing. Three tablespoons of ranch dressing has 17 grams of fat and calories. That's 87 percent of calories from fat, more fat than 4 ounces of vanilla ice cream and more calories than ½ cup of flan or a serving of tortilla chips and salsa. Experiment with low- or non-fat dressings until you find one you you and the kids enjoy.

Movie snacks are loaded with trouble. One small box of popcorn with "butter" topping turns a low-cal treat into a 200–400-calorie, fat-soaked no-no. Skip the topping. One ounce of peanut M&Ms weighs in with 45 percent of its 143 calories from fat! (And you never, never eat just 1 ounce.) Pass up the candy.

Prepared spaghetti sauces. In a ½ cup of some extra-thick zesty tomato sauces, a whopping 96 percent of the calories are from fat. But many healthy choices have no fat at all. Read labels and compare.

Condiments. Creamy dips and toppings can turn a lean meal into a fat feast. Tartar sauce has 8 grams of fat a tablespoon. Real mayonnaise is loaded with eggs and oil: It has 10 fat grams a tablespoon—almost one-quarter of all the fat many of us should have in a day. Imitation mayo brings the fat down to 2 to 4 grams a tablespoon.

Margarine is not so good. It's 100 percent fat and, although it contains no cholesterol, solidified vegetable oil contains transfats that keep the body from clearing out excess cholesterol. On toast, try substituting apple butter—no fat, lots of flavor!

Salad bars are potential trouble spots because you assume you're eating healthful foods. In fact, 3 tablespoons of shredded cheddar cheese adds 7 grams of fat; ½ cup coleslaw adds 8 grams; 2 tablespoons egg = 2 grams of fat; 2 tablespoons of bacon bits = 3 grams fat; and 1 packet or 2½ ounces of blue cheese dressing weighs in with 34 grams of fat. Your salad has gone from no fat and few calories, to 54 grams of fat and 600 calories—more than all the fat and one-third of the calories you should have in a day if you don't exercise regularly.

Just a little milk in your coffee? Two tablespoons of cream has 9 grams fat; 2 tablespoons of half-and-half has 3.6 grams fat; ¼ cup of whole milk has 2.1 grams; skim milk has almost no fat.

How to Change
Your Eating Habits

The best way to start a healthy diet is to wean yourself slowly off higher-fat, less-nutritious foods. Take the time to find low-fat substitutes that you enjoy eating. And remember, if you're going to give up fat, you don't have to give up other treats as well. Real Vermont maple syrup doesn't have any fat. Neither does strawberry jam or yummy orange sorbet. Give up hot fudge sundaes—but go for an occasional orange sorbet covered in orange marmalade! It has no fat at all!

Getting Started

At home, make sure you use cholesterol-free, monounsaturated oils such as olive oil. Monounsaturated oils help lower bad cholesterol (LDLs), which causes heart disease, and increase good cholesterol (HDL). Avoid cooking with animal fats such as lard.

And no frying. Put olive oil in a spray bottle and use it to lightly coat pans or flavor vegetables before cooking.

Eat breakfast every day—one piece of fruit and/or a glass of juice; cereal with low-fat milk; whole grain toast. Studies indicate that people who eat a healthy breakfast lose weight more effectively and control their cholesterol.

Always have a steamed or fresh vegetable with lunch and dinner (catsup is not a vegetable). The fiber in vegetables appears to help fight heart disease and the phytochemicals are thought to fight cancer.

Smart vs. Not-So-Smart Choices

Fish sticks: 3 ounces = 228 calories; 41 percent of
calories from fat

vs.

Baked haddock: 3 ounces = 95 calories; 7 percent of
calories from fat

Bologna: 1 ounce = 90 calories; 80 percent of calories
from fat

vs.

Turkey breast: 1 ounce = 86 calories; 5 percent of
calories from fat

Fried chicken: 6–7 ounces = 532 calories; 53 percent of
calories from fat
dark meat with skin

vs.

Roasted chicken: 6–7 ounces = 242 calories; 22 percent
of calories from fat
white meat, no skin

Drink to Your Health

Your body needs at least 64 ounces of fresh water a day. And
you are better off with no caffeine, from coffee or colas. Although the health risks of caffeine are reported to be minimal,
those who rely heavily on the drug are depleting their energy,
developing a dependency on a stimulant, and often engage in
other unhealthy habits, such as getting insufficient sleep,
smoking, and drinking too much alcohol. While you're spa-

Cutting Out the Caffeine

If you want to remove caffeine from your diet, it's best to back off slowly. Going cold turkey produces terrible headaches and generally doesn't work since the rewards of having a cup of joe are immediate and the harm seems so minimal. Instead, The Wellness Center recommends gradual withdrawal over the course of four to five weeks.

Week One: Drink coffee as you usually do, only write down the time whenever you have a cup. You may be surprised how much you drink in the course of the day. Figure out how many cups, on average, you drink a day.

Week Two: Eliminate 1 cup a day if you drink 4 cups or less a day.

Eliminate 2 cups a day if you drink 5 or more cups a day.

Week Three: If you are currently drinking 2 cups a day, reduce intake to 1 cup caffeinated coffee a day and no more than 2 cups of decaf.

ing, try to cut caffeine to the minimum needed to avoid a caffeine withdrawal headache. And then make a promise to yourself to try the coffee withdrawal plan above.

Pyramid Power

The simplest way to change the types and quantities of food you eat is to follow the new Food Pyramid. This system, developed by the U.S. Department of Agriculture, replaces the

If you are currently drinking 3 or more cups a day, reduce intake to 2 cups of caffeinated coffee a day and no more than 1 cup of decaf.

Week Four: If you are currently drinking 1 cup of high test and 2 cups of decaf a day, make every other day an all-decaf day.

If you are currently drinking 2 cups of high test a day and 1 cup of decaf, switch so that you're drinking 1 cup of high test and 2 cups of decaf.

Week Five: Those of you who have been making every other day a decaf day, are ready to go all decaf. For those of you who are now down to one cup of high test a day, make every other day an all-decaf day.

Week Six: You should be all decaf now. You'll be stunned how often you leave the house in the morning without bothering to make a cup of decaf coffee. It simply becomes irrelevant—you start off your day with plenty of energy and no need for an artificial boost of caffeine.

old Four Basic Food Groups. If you follow it, you will automatically be on a low-fat nutritious diet.

What's a Serving?
- Oils and fats should be limited to 5 to 8 servings a day, including fats in prepared foods. 1 serving = 1 tsp. vegetable oil or margarine; 1 T. salad dressing; 2 tsp. mayonnaise; 3 tsp. seeds or nuts; 1/8 of an avocado; 10 small olives
- Milk, yogurt, or cheese: 1 serving = 1 c. milk or yogurt and 1.5 to 2 ozs. cheese

Fats, Oils,
Sweets
use sparingly

Milk,   Meat, Poultry, Fish,
Yogurt, Cheese   Dry Beans, Nuts, Eggs
2–3 servings daily   *2–3 servings daily*

Vegetables   Fruit
3–5 servings daily   *2–4 servings daily*

Bread   Rice   Cereals   Pasta
                   6–11 servings daily

- Vegetables: 1 serving = ½ c. chopped vegetables or 1 c. leafy raw vegetables
- Fruits: 1 serving = ¾ c. juice, ½ c. canned fruit, 1 piece of fruit or a melon wedge, ¼ c. dried fruit
- Meat, poultry, fish: 1 serving = 2.5 to 3 ozs.
- One egg, ½ c. cooked beans, or 2 T. peanut butter = ⅓ a serving
- Breads, cereals, rice and pasta: 1 serving = 1 slice bread, ½ c. cooked rice or pasta, ½ c. cooked cereal, 1 oz. cold cereal

Sources—The FDA Consumer Special Report: Focus on Food Labeling;
The American Heart Association: An Eating Plan for Healthy Americans.

How Much Should You Eat?

How many servings a day you should eat depends on your age and amount of daily activity. All recommendations are designed to maintain your weight. For weight loss, eat the

Sample Daily Diets for Women

	LOW ACTIVITY LEVEL OR WEIGHT LOSS (1,600 CALORIES A DAY)	MODERATE ACTIVITY LEVEL (2,200 CALORIES A DAY)
Bread group servings	6	9
Vegetable group	3	4
Fruit group servings	2	2–3
Milk group servings	2–3*	2–3
Meat group ounces	5	6

Total Protein: 44 grams for women (average woman eats 60); 60 grams for pregnant women

*Pregnant or breast-feeding women and young women ages 11–24 need 3–4 servings from the milk group.
Sources: National Research Council and USDA.

same number of servings but choose lower-calorie foods, and don't go below 1,200 to 1,400 calories a day.

Foods That Fight Disease

We are constantly flooded with extravagant claims about the health-giving benefits of specific vitamins or foods. But much of the evidence is inconclusive, and it's hard to know exactly how much of a food, vitamin, or mineral to consume to get the claimed effect. To clear up the confusion, the USDA, the FDA, and the Surgeon General have investigated a wide variety of claims. Their conclusions:

Calcium-rich Foods and Osteoporosis

The calcium in dairy products, leafy green vegetables, and some seafood does help prevent osteoporosis, the weakening of bones that hits many women after menopause. Osteopo-

Sources of Calcium

Yogurt	8 ounces, low-fat, plain	415 mg
Skim milk	1 cup	302 mg
Swiss cheese	1 ounce	272 mg
Sardines	2 ounces	250 mg
Broccoli	½ cup fresh	79 mg
Oranges	1 medium	55 mg
Green beans	½ cup fresh	31 mg

rosis causes about 1.3 million bone fractures a year. The National Research Council recommends that children between 1 and 10 take in 800 mg a day. From ages 11 to 24 the need goes up to 1,200 mg. Women 25 or older need 800 mg and pregnant women need 1,200 mg. The National Dairy Board points out, however, that many experts believe that women should consume 1,000 to 1,500 mg before menopause in order to make their bones strong enough to avoid osteoporosis. Furthermore, they suggest that after menopause women on estrogen therapy should take in 1,000 mg calcium. Those not on estrogen therapy should take in 1,500. But don't overdo it! Exceeding recommended levels can cause bone pain, digestive upset, kidney stones, and disorientation.

Fiber-filled Foods, Heart Disease and Cancer

Fruits, vegetables, and grain products that contain fiber appear to reduce the risk of cancer—the Surgeon General has said they may be particularly effective in preventing colorectal cancer. And the FDA says that fruit, vegetables, and grain products that contain fiber may reduce the risk of coronary heart disease by reducing cholesterol levels.

The National Cancer Institute recommends that we eat between 20 and 35 grams of fiber a day, but the average American only eats 10 grams. The best way to increase your daily dose is to add shredded wheat, rolled oats (oatmeal), dried

Sources of Fiber

Grams of fiber per 100 grams (about 3 ounces) of food:

WATER SOLUBLE	WATER INSOLUBLE
Dry oat bran 7.2g	All-bran 24.9g
Dried white beans 1.7g	Shredded wheat 10.2g
Dried split peas 1.6g	Barley 7.4g
Cooked rolled oats .8g	Asparagus 2.8g
Strawberries .8g	Brussels sprouts 2.7g
Apples .7g	Green beans 2.3g
Bananas .6g	Carrots 1.9g
	Broccoli 1.7g

beans, and a wide variety of fruits and vegetables to your diet. That will give you enough water-soluble fiber (which reduces cholesterol and stabilizes blood sugar levels) and insoluble fiber (which aids the digestive tract).

Vitamin A and Cancer

Foods with high levels of vitamin A and beta-carotene, such as dark green leafy vegetables, deep yellow vegetables, tomatoes, and dairy products, may help prevent lung, bladder, and oral cavity cancers, says the 1988 Surgeon General's Report on Nutrition and Health. Other studies show that vitamin A may help cut the risk of breast cancer.

What About Vitamin Supplements?

Americans spend around $3,000,000,000 (that's three billion!) a year on vitamin supplements. But you can't buy health in a bottle. Nothing can take the place of a balanced diet that provides all the nutrients your body needs. However, taking a multiple vitamin that provides about 150 percent of the daily recommended amounts may be helpful and surely won't hurt.

Cut Back on Meat

Studies by the National Cancer Institute show that women who eat two to three servings of meat a day are twice as likely to suffer from endometrial cancer as women who eat less meat. And the Harvard Nurses Study of more than 88,000 people found that if you eat red meat four or more times a week, you double your chances of developing colon cancer.

If you choose to take higher doses of vitamins, remember they are made to work together—taking a high dose of one may throw other vitamins and minerals out of whack. Furthermore, at high levels some vitamins and minerals are toxic. More is not always better.

FDA's Recommended Daily Intake

Vitamin A | 5,000 IU From dairy, green leafy and yellow vegetables.

Vitamin C | 60 mg Available in fruits and vegetables.

Thiamin (B1) | 1.5 mg Available in unrefined grains and rice, legumes, and green leafy vegetables.

Riboflavin (B2) | 1.7 mg Available in fish, whole grains, and green leafy vegetables.

Niacin (B3) | 20 mg Available in fish, yeast, whole grains, dried peas, beans, and nuts.

Calcium | 800 mg Available in dairy products, green leafy vegetables, and some seafood.

Protect Your Heart

Recent studies suggest that vitamin E and beta-carotene (a form of vitamin A) may help keep LDL cholesterol from sticking to artery walls. These vitamins are called antioxidants. For vitamin A, the best sources are carrots, kale, sweet red peppers, spinach, winter squash, sweet potatoes, turnip greens, oatmeal, and mangoes.

Foods high in vitamin E: greens, especially chard, dandelion, mustard, and turnip; apples, apricots; fortified ready-to-eat cereals; mullet, perch, salmon, scallops, shrimp; nuts such as almonds and filberts; sunflower seeds.

Iron	18 mg Available in lean meat, shellfish, dried beans, fruits, whole grains, green leafy vegetables, and blackstrap molasses. (It's as bad to have too much as too little.)
Vitamin D	400 IU Available from sunshine, oily fish.
Vitamin E	30 IU Available from wheat germ oil; oils from cereal grains, such as soybean, cottonseed, sunflower, and corn oil; nuts, eggs, and fish.
Vitamin B6	2.0 mg Available in whole grain cereals, wheat germ, soybeans, yeast, peanuts, corn, and blackstrap molasses.
Folic Acid	.4 mg Available in dark green leafy vegetables, asparagus, lima beans, whole grains, lentils, and orange juice.
Vitamin B12	6 mcg Available in meat, fish, and milk.
Phosphorus	1.0 g Available in meat, fish, poultry, eggs, milk, cheese, nuts, and legumes
Iodine	150 mcg Available in iodized salt, seafood, and kelp.

Magnesium	400 mg Available in legumes, nuts, whole grains, and shellfish.
Zinc	5 mg Available in oysters, herring, meats, dairy, eggs, and legumes.
Copper	2 mg Available in nuts, mushrooms, seafood, chocolate, and legumes.
Biotin	.3 mg Available in egg yolks, peanuts, mushrooms, cauliflower, and whole grains.
Pantothenic acid	10 mg Available in peanuts, broccoli, cauliflower, whole grains, and bran.

Sources: FDA and National Academy of Sciences RDA's.

Test Your Nutrition IQ

1. What contains the most fat?
   a) one ounce of cream cheese
   b) McDonald's Quarter Pounder
   c) one avocado

2. Which vegetables usually have the most vitamins?
   a) canned
   b) frozen
   c) fresh

3. Which is best for you?
   a) olive oil
   b) canola oil
   c) solid margarine
   d) lard

4. Fiber is found in:
   a) strawberries
   b) pork chops
   c) sardines

5. There is more cholesterol in:
   a) one stick of margarine
   b) ¼ pound shrimp
   c) ½ a broiled chicken breast, no skin

6. Calcium is found in:
   a) sardines
   b) cheese
   c) kale
   d) all of the above

7. Cholesterol is found in:
   a) all fatty foods
   b) vegetables
   c) meat, fish, and poultry

8. You need to eat:
   a) at least 6 servings of rice, pasta, or bread a day
   b) 2–3 servings of fruit a day
   c) 2–3 servings of vegetables a day
   d) all of the above

9. Which has more fat:
   a) a lean three-ounce hamburger or
   b) a salad with 3 tablespoons of Italian dressing on it?

10. Many women don't take in:
    a) enough calcium to keep their bones from becoming brittle in old age
    b) enough fiber to combat digestive problems
    c) a balanced diet, which may help fight breast cancer
    d) all of the above

Answers:

1. An avocado. It has 30 g of fat—about half of most people's daily allotment—not what you had in mind

when you enjoyed that guacamole last night. An ounce of cream cheese has 9.9 g and the Quarter Pounder, 20.7 g. (To its credit, an avocado has no cholesterol, not much saturated fat, and a good dose of monounsaturated fat—which cannot be said for either the Quarter Pounder or the cream cheese.)

2. Frozen. Most fresh vegetables sit around for days and days after they are picked, losing vitamins at a steady clip. Frozen vegetables are processed less than 6 hours after picking, sealing in 50 to 90 percent of the vitamins.

3. Olive oil. It has 10 grams of monounsaturated fat in one tablespoon; canola oil has around 8, while lard has less than 6 and margarine only 4. Overall each has between 11 and 14 grams of fat per tablespoon.

4. Strawberries. Fiber is found in fruits, vegetables, and grains. It can help keep your digestive tract healthy, may lower cholesterol, and reduces the risk of heart disease and cancer.

5. Shrimp. It has 221 milligrams of cholesterol; ½ breast of skinless chicken has only 73, and margarine has none. You should limit your cholesterol intake to 300 mgs a day!

6. All of the above. Women need at least 800 mg of calcium a day (ages 11–24 require 1,200 mg) but almost none of us meet the minimum daily requirement. If we drank two glasses of skim milk a day (604 mg of calcium), we'd go a long way toward fighting osteoporosis—the disease that makes older women stoop-shouldered and susceptible to broken bones.

7. Meat, fish, and poultry. Cholesterol is found only in animal products.

Information Please!

For general information on nutrition write for

Dietary Guidelines and Your Diet and
Nutritive Values of Foods
Human Nutrition Information Service USDA,
Room 325DA
6505 Belcrest Road
Hyattsville, MD 20782

Eating for Your Life and other publications
National Institutes of Health, Room 10 A 24
Building 31
Bethesda, MD 20892

8. All of the above. For more information, see the Food Pyramid on page 172.
9. The salad—once you pour on the dressing!
10. All of the above! But women can improve their health if they change the types and quantities of foods they eat. Remember, you *can* take charge of your well-being.

Spa Recipes

·

The recipes contained in this section are designed to show you just how easy it is to integrate healthful dishes into your everyday meals. We present basic suggestions for fruit, vegetable, and meat recipes and then suggest how to vary them slightly, so that you can use them for snacks, main courses, or a light lunch.

Fruit and Vegetable Juices

Natural fruit juices are a great source of fiber when the pulp is not filtered out. And they are rich in vitamin C—a glass of carrot juice offers 475 percent of the recommended daily allowance and orange juice has 200 percent. B vitamins are in good supply in tomato juice—particularly folic acid—and vegetable juice cocktail has 21 percent of the RDA for vitamin A. All with no fat and few calories. In addition to fresh juices available at your health food store, you may want to try these tasty beverages:

Fresh Fruit Frappes

♦

You can enjoy this as a breakfast drink, an afternoon pick-me-up, or a cooler anytime of day. Try one in the tub as you soak in a lovely herbal spa treatment.

1 cup fresh berries
½ cup crushed ice
½ cup unsweetened fruit juice (orange, pineapple, mango, papaya)
½ cup club soda

*a touch of herbs can make the fruit frappe an integral part
    of your spa treatment.*

To make the drink invigorating:

add 1 teaspoon grated fresh ginger

To make it calming:

add ½ cup chamomile tea (at room temperature)

To make it provocative:

add 1–2 tablespoons chopped fresh peppermint leaves

Combine ingredients in blender, adding ice and juice until desired consistency is reached.

Serves 2

Calories: 97 Fat: less than 1 gram Carbohydrates: 22 grams
Protein: less than 2 grams Cholesterol: 0

Smoothies Plus

◆

These make great diet lunches during a spa weekend or anytime you're trying to keep your energy high and your fat intake
extra low.

> *1 cup orange juice*
> *1 ripe banana*
> *½ cup skim milk*
> *dash of vanilla*
> *ice*

Combine ingredients in blender, adding ice (or more
juice) to reach desired consistency.

You may change around the recipe by adding any unsweetened fruit juice or fresh fruits.

And to fortify a smoothie—a good idea if you're using it

as a meal—add brewer's yeast, wheat germ, protein mix, or low-fat yogurt.

Calories: 267 Fat: 1–2 grams Carbohydrates: 73 grams
Protein: 8 grams Cholesterol: 0

Vegetable Drinks

•

If you don't have a juicer, you can still make vegetable drinks by relying on leafy greens and tomatoes.

2 fresh tomatoes
1 cup fresh spinach, arugula, and buttercup lettuce
horseradish
tobasco
salt and pepper to taste

In a blender combine tomatoes, chopped, with lightly steamed, cooled fresh spinach, arugula, and buttercup lettuce. Blend well.

Add tobasco, horseradish, pepper, and a dash of salt to taste.

Serve over ice garnished with a celery or carrot stick. Or you could have had a low-sodium V-8.

Calories: 80 Fat: 1 gram Carbohydrates: 16 grams
Protein: 4 grams Cholesterol: 0

Fruit and Vegetable Side Dishes and Entrées

Luscious Fruit Salad

◆

½ cup each of:
diced oranges
halved green grapes
sliced bananas
cubed mangoes

whole or halved berries
chunks of cantaloupe or
    other melon
juice of ½ lime
½ tsp cinnamon

Toss fruit with lime juice and cinnamon. Stir. Serve at room temperature.

Serves 3

PER SERVING—Calories: 90 Carbohydrates: 21 grams
Protein: 1.5 grams Cholesterol: 0 milligrams Fat: .5 grams

Rice-Fruit Salad

◆

To basic fruit salad, above, add:
2 cups cold, cooked rice (brown or white) seasoned with ¼ cup raisins (optional), 1–2 tablespoons chopped cilantro or Italian parsley, ½–1 teaspoon rosemary leaves, diced and crushed, and 1–2 tablespoons olive oil. Taste, adjust seasoning.

Serve at room temperature with warm pita.

Serves 6

PER SERVING—Calories: 218 Carbohydrates: 41 grams
Protein: 3 grams Cholesterol: 0 milligrams Fat: 5.5 grams

Sweet Treat

◆

Fruit salad dessert:
Line large glass bowl with low-fat ladyfingers. Spread half the basic fruit salad over the cookies. (You may want to increase the amount of banana for this variation.) Smooth a layer of 1 cup low-fat or nonfat plain yogurt over fruit. Top with a sprinkling of crumbled cookie crumbs. Cover with remaining fruit. Garnish with yogurt and chopped mint. Let sit for no more than 30 minutes. Serve at room temperature.

Serves 6

PER SERVING—Calories: 60 Carbohydrates: 43 grams
Protein: 5.5 grams Cholesterol: 108 milligrams Fat: 3.5 grams

Veggie Deluxe

◆

Using a basic recipe for steamed vegetables with a low-fat yogurt sauce, you can create a pasta dinner or a wonderful tuna salad.

10 thin spears of asparagus
½ cup green beans
½ cup snap peas
1 cup broccoli spears
5 pickled onions
1 tablespoon capers
4 artichoke hearts (not in oil), or any other prepared
    veggies you like

For the sauce:
½ cup low-fat plain yogurt
2 tablespoons fresh dill
½ cucumber, peeled, seeded
pepper

Steam or parboil all veggies except cucumber until cooked but crunchy. Arrange on platter with onions, capers, and artichoke hearts.

Mix together yogurt, dill, and cucumber sliced paper-thin. Add a dash of pepper. Serve as dipping sauce or pour over vegetables.

Serves 2–4

PER SERVING (FROM TOTAL OF 4 SERVINGS)—
Calories: 87 Carbohydrates: 15 grams Protein: 7 grams
Cholesterol: 7 milligrams Fat: 1 gram

. . . *with pasta*

♦

Cook ⅔ cup small shells or bow tie pasta. Drain and cool. Toss with vegetable yogurt mixture above. Serve at room temperature.

Serves 4

Calories: 140 Carbohydrates: 26 grams Protein: 9 grams
Cholesterol: 7 milligrams Fat: 1 gram

. . . with fish

•

Fill a large salad bowl with 1–2 cups mixed organic field greens (or your favorite lettuce). Sprinkle with 1 can white tuna in water, drained. Toss in veggie-yogurt recipe from above. Serve.

Serves 3

Calories: 130 Carbohydrates: 16 grams Protein: 15 grams
Cholesterol: 12 milligrams Fat: 1 gram

Beans and Legumes

An essential part of any healthy diet, beans and legumes are, for many Americans, an undiscovered culinary treat. Beyond refried beans, way beyond lard-laced baked beans, are the exotic flavors of beans found in Italian, Japanese, and Mexican cooking.

Besides being fiber-rich and cholesterol-lowering, a half a cup is packed with nutrients:

Japanese adzuki beans	70% RDA folic acid	23% RDA iron	29 grams carbohydrates	147 calories 0 grams fat
Black beans	64% RDA folic acid	18% RDA iron	20 grams carbohydrates	114 calories 0 grams fat
Kidney beans	57% RDA folic acid	26% RDA iron	20 grams carbohydrates	112 calories 0 grams fat
Lentils	89% RDA folic acid	33% RDA iron	20 grams carbohydrates	115 calories 0 grams fat

Black Bean Bonanza

◆

1 can black beans, not drained
½ teaspoon cinnamon (or more to taste)
hot sauce

Simmer beans with cinnamon and hot sauce to taste, until most of the liquid has evaporated and beans are soft but not mushy.

Serve on an oven-toasted (no oil) corn or flour tortilla. Top with chopped onions, tomatoes, cilantro, green peppers, and/or asparagus spears. Garnish with tomato salsa or mango salsa.

Serves 2

PER SERVING—Calories: 265 Carbohydrates: 43 grams
Protein: 12 grams Cholesterol: 0 grams Fat: 2.5 grams

Tuscan Bean Salad

◆

This cold salad is delicious served on mesclun salad greens and topped with a sprinkle of fresh reggianno parmesan.

1 can drained white cannellini beans
2 cloves garlic, diced
1 tablespoon fresh lemon juice
3 stalks celery, chopped fine
fresh Italian parsley
1 tablespoon olive oil
dash pepper

Mix and adjust seasoning to taste. Spoon onto a bed of lettuce. Top with tablespoon of fresh, grated parmesan.

Serves 4

PER SERVING—Calories: 170 Carbohydrates: 18 grams
Protein: 7 grams Cholesterol: 4 milligrams Fat: 6 grams

Scrumptious Sauces

The key to wonderful low-fat healthy food is a good sauce that keeps you from pining for fried foods, buttery sauces, and mayonnaise-based condiments.

The following sauces offer a range of flavors and textures, and can be used on rice, pasta, chicken, fish, or veggies.

Mango Salsa

♦

Great served at room temperature with chicken, fish, veggies, or pasta. Also can be used to baste fish and chicken when broiled or grilled.

1 ripe mango
½ sweet onion
2 large tomatoes
1 tablespoon chopped cilantro
juice of ½ fresh lime
2 tablespoons orange juice
cayenne pepper to taste

Dice the mango, onion, and tomatoes. Place half of them in a blender. Add juice of ½ fresh lime and orange juice. Add cayenne pepper to taste. Blend for about 10 seconds, until well mixed but not entirely smooth.

Combine with the remaining half of the unblended ingredients. Sprinkle with chopped cilantro.

PER TABLESPOON—Calories: 14 Carbohydrates: 4 grams
Protein: 0 grams Cholesterol: 0 milligrams Fat: 0 grams

Ancho Chili Sauce

♦

This tomato-based sauce relies on the smoky flavor of the ancho chili for its distinctive flavor. Mix with rice or pasta; use to baste broiled skinless chicken breasts.

1 whole dried ancho chili
10 cherry tomatoes
1 tablespoon olive oil
3 cloves garlic, chopped fine
½ onion, diced
2 tablespoons fat-free chicken broth
2 tablespoons chopped cilantro (optional)

Place ancho chili on a long grilling fork and hold over open flame on gas range. Allow it to flame up very briefly on each side. Then cut off top and remove seeds from inside. Chop chili and set aside. If you don't have an open flame available, use the broiler set at top temperature.

In a small, heavy frying pan combine olive oil, onion, garlic. Sauté over low heat until onions are translucent and sweet. Add chopped ancho chili and cook for 2 minutes.

Add chicken broth and cherry tomatoes, cut in half.

Stir often and press tomatoes to release juices. Keep temperature low so juice does not boil away. Add cilantro just before serving.

PER TABLESPOON—Calories: 25 Carbohydrates: 2 grams
Protein: 0 grams Cholesterol: 0 milligrams Fat: 2 grams

Garlic Basil Sauce

◆

Spread on vegetables or chicken before grilling, or mix into mashed potatoes or pasta.

> *1 large garlic bulb*
> *1–2 tablespoons olive oil*
> *¼ cup chopped fresh basil leaves (optional—you can omit, or substitute any herb you fancy)*

Coat the garlic bulb with olive oil.

Place in covered clay dish or wrap in aluminum foil.

Roast in 325°F oven until tender—about 20 minutes.

When it's done, press all the softened garlic out of the cloves and mix in a bowl with 1–2 tablespoons olive oil and finely chopped basil.

Stir in 1 tablespoon per serving of pasta. Garnish with fresh basil leaves and a light dusting of parmesan.

PER TABLESPOON—Calories: 30 Carbohydrates: 3 grams
Protein: 0 grams Cholesterol: 0 milligrams Fat: 7 grams

Balsamic Basting Sauce

◆

Balsamic vinegar can be used straight from the bottle to baste, grill, or broil fresh vegetables and as a tasty salad dressing. It is also good on broiled, skinless chicken. (The chicken in this book is always served skinless, but we didn't need to tell you that, now, did we?) If the flavor of the vinegar is somewhat strong for you, add a dash of sugar, or a tablespoon of orange marmalade, to every ¼ cup.

And the calories aren't even worth mentioning.

Marinara Sauce

◆

A basic tomato sauce that's sweet and full of pure flavors and goes with everything from rice and beans to tuna fish and pasta.

3 cloves garlic, diced
1 tablespoon olive oil
1 sweet onion, chopped fine
1 large can whole Italian tomatoes with basil

Place olive oil in a heavy frying pan.

Add diced garlic and onion.

Sauté over low flame until onion and garlic begin to brown. If they stick to the pan, add a tablespoon or two of low-fat chicken broth.

Add one large can whole Italian tomatoes, cut into small chunks.

Simmer over low heat for five to ten minutes, stirring frequently. Taste. Add pepper, a dash of salt. Keep flavors simple and pure and allow the sweetness of the tomatoes to dominate.

Serve over pasta or use as liquid for steamed fish, or as a marinade for stewed chicken.

Serves 4

PER SERVING—Calories: 50 Carbohydrates: 4 grams
Protein: 0 grams Cholesterol: 0 milligrams Fat: 4 grams

Fish and Meat

Fish Fantastic

•

For the very best-tasting, low-calorie fish dishes, nothing cooks like a parchment paper pouch. You can buy a roll of the parchment paper at the grocery store or food specialty shop.

2 halibut steaks, ½ pound each
1 recipe of mango salsa (see page 193)
¼ pound snow pea pods

Tear off 2 parchment sheets about 12 inches long. Place a halibut steak in the middle of each sheet.

Spoon about ¼ cup of mango salsa around the fish and over the top.

Place about 8–10 snow peas around the fish, on top of the salsa.

Seal the parchment by bringing the edges to the center and then folding them over together to make a tight seam. Seal the ends by twisting the parchment tightly and then folding it upward and tucking it under itself. There must not be any gaps or openings in the package.

Place parchment packages in a large sheet cake pan and cook at 500°F for about 10–20 minutes, depending on thickness of fish steak. (You can check if it's ready by opening a pouch after 10 minutes and poking fish with fork.)

Be careful opening the packages because steam will burn you. Serve with extra salsa.

To vary the recipe, add one of the other sauces from above, a variety of vegetables, and/or different types of fish. If you use delicate fish such as filet of sole, choose a light-flavored sauce and steam for 10 minutes. You can also top the filets with three fresh shrimp (in or out of shells). They will cook along with the fish. (That adds 45 calories, 83 milligrams of cholesterol, and 9 grams of protein.)

Serves 2

PER SERVING—Calories: 296 Carbohydrates:18 grams
Protein: 45 grams Cholesterol: 70 milligrams Fat: 5 grams

Best Roast Chicken Ever

◆

Using a free-range; organic chicken, remove all the skin and extra fat that accumulates near the opening to the insides.

Slather the chicken with Dijon or coarse ground mustard.

Preheat the oven to 500°F.

Place chicken in a heavy cast-iron skillet or heavy-duty low-sided pan.

Cook until done, about 50 minutes to an hour for a 3.5-pound bird.

Chicken is done with there is no pink around the second joint and the juices run clear.

PER 3 OZ. SERVING WHITE MEAT, NO SKIN (for dark meat add 9 calories, 2 grams of fat, and 9 milligrams of cholesterol to figures)—
Calories: 142 Carbohydrates: 0 grams Protein: 27 grams
Cholesterol: 73 milligrams Fat: 3 grams

Sweet and Spicy Beef Salad

◆

6 ounces lean, hormone-free beef, sliced thin
¼ cup low-sodium soy sauce
1 teaspoon sugar
1 teaspoon red pepper flakes
¼ cup sherry
pinch of grated ginger root
1 cup organic mesclun mix or bib and romaine lettuce

Remove all fat from meat and slice into very thin strips about 1½ inches long.

Combine other ingredients and pour over meat. Let marinate for 20 minutes.

Heat a heavy skillet or wok until it almost smokes.

Drain and save juices from the beef.

Add beef to hot wok. Stir often, tossing pieces in pan. When cooked medium rare, add juice. Keep stirring for another minute at most.

Serve over organic field greens as a dinner salad.

Serves 2

PER SERVING—Calories: 211 Carbohydrates: 0 grams
Protein: 26 grams Cholesterol: 76 milligrams Fat: 6 grams

Spa Breakfasts

One more thing Mama was right about: Breakfast *is* the most important meal of the day. Study after study has revealed that how you eat in the morning affects your metabolism all day long—in fact, skipping breakfast can make you gain, not lose, weight and set you up for a major mid-afternoon energy sink.

The goal is to eat no less than a third and no more than half of your day's calories in your morning meal. For those on 1,600-calorie-a-day diets that means between 535 and 800 calories. On a 2,200-calorie diet, it comes to between 735 and 1,100. See the chart at right where we've listed some of the healthiest and tastiest breakfast foods—mix and match them to suit your tastes and calorie requirements.

The Spa Menus

In the following spa menus, we set out spa-healthy breakfasts, lunches, and dinners for you to enjoy during your at-home spa sessions. These meals can also serve as a general guide for the kinds of foods and flavors you can integrate into your everyday cuisine. Long on flavor and short on fat and calories, they will help you and your family feel and look younger and more vibrant.

	CALORIES	FAT	CARBOHYDRATES	PROTEIN	CHOLESTEROL
BREADS					
English muffin	155	1g	30g	5g	0mg
Whole wheat bread—1 oz.	70	>1g	13g	2g	0mg
Large bagel	235	3g	60g	12g	0mg
Pita bread	105	>1g	21g	4g	
CEREALS					
1 cup oatmeal, cooked	110	2g	18g	4g	0mg
1 large shredded wheat	80	>1g			0mg
1 cup corn flakes	100	0g			0mg
FRUITS					
½ cantaloupe	58	>1g	14g	1g	0mg
10 strawberries	45	>1g	11g	1g	0mg
Banana	105	>1g	27g	1g	0mg
Papaya	60	>1	15g	> 1	0mg
Apple	85	>1	21g	> 1g	0mg
½ grapefruit	40	>1	10g	> 1g	0mg
JUICES					
4 oz. orange	56	>1	13g	1g	0mg
4 oz. grapefruit	50	>1	22g	1g	0mg
4 oz. apple	58	>1g	15g	> 1g	0mg
4 oz. cranberry	72	>1g	18g	0g	0mg
4 oz. tomato	20	>1g	4g	> 1g	0mg

> = less than

Goals

20–30% of calories from fat = 31–53 grams of fat
300 to 250 milligrams cholesterol
5 servings fresh vegetables (2.5 cups cooked)
3 servings fruit (3 pieces)
8 servings of grains, rice, and legumes
2 servings dairy (2 cups milk or yogurt)
no more than 6 ounces of meat, fish, or poultry

For a 1,200–1,600-Calorie Day

This is an austere diet, for weight loss under supervision of a
nutritionist or doctor.

*Breakfast target: maximum of 500 calories and
10 grams of fat*

MENU
8 ounces orange juice
1 banana
1 large shredded wheat
½ cup skim milk
1 slice wheat toast
1 tablespoon honey
3 glasses of water between breakfast and lunch

Total: 481 calories, 3 grams fat, 5 milligrams cholesterol; 1½
fruit servings, 3 grain servings, 1 dairy serving

Lunch target: maximum of 400 calories and 10 grams of fat

MENU

1 serving Tuscan bean salad (page 192)

3 ounces roast skinless chicken, white or dark meat

½ cup steamed rice with herbs

1 glass skim milk

1 cup fruit salad

3 glasses of water between lunch- and dinnertime

Total: 402 calories, 9.5 grams fat, 73 milligrams cholesterol; 3 rice and legume servings, 2 fruit servings, 1 meat serving

Optional Snack target: maximum of 300 calories and a trace of fat

MENU

2 servings fresh vegetables and yogurt dill dip (page 189)

1 toasted pita bread

1 glass tomato juice

Total: 310 calories, 1 gram fat; 3 vegetable servings, 1 grain serving, ½ dairy serving

Dinner target: (with snack) 300 calories and 17 grams of fat; (without snack) 500 calories and 17 grams of fat

300-CALORIE DINNER

1 serving sweet and spicy beef salad (see page 199)

1 glass skim milk

3 glasses of water between dinner and bedtime

Total: 311 calories, 6 grams fat, 80 milligrams cholesterol; 1 meat serving, 1 dairy serving, 2 vegetable servings

500-Calorie Dinner

◆

1 serving steamed halibut (page 197)

1 baked potato—with either nonfat sour cream or yogurt,
*   or spicy salsa*

1 tossed salad with balsamic oil-free dressing

1 glass skim milk

3 glasses of water between dinner and bedtime

Total: 541 calories, 5 grams fat, 85 milligrams cholesterol; 2½
meat servings, 2 vegetable servings, 1–1½ dairy servings

This diet is very low in fat with around 25 grams for the day and less than 200 milligrams of cholesterol: good for the heart and for weight loss, but difficult—and in almost all cases, unnecessary—to maintain. Even with such a low level of fat, you do meet the recommended daily intake of food groups: You get 2½ servings of fruit and dairy, 5–7 servings of grain, 7 of vegetables, and 2–2½ of meat. And calories are very low, too, although you come in at 1,480 with the snack and beef salad—slightly over the goal. But don't eat less. Simply take an after-dinner stroll for about 30 minutes.

Goals

20–30% of calories from fat = 44–66 grams fat
250 milligrams cholesterol
5 servings fresh vegetables (2.5 cups cooked)
3 servings fruit (3 pieces)
8 servings of grains, rice, and legumes
2 servings dairy (2 cups milk or yogurt)
no more than 2 servings of meat, fish, or poultry (4–6
   ounces a day)

For an 1,800–2,000-Calorie Day

*Breakfast target: maximum 500 calories and 5–10
grams of fat*

MENU
½ papaya
1 English muffin
1 bowl of corn flakes
½ cup milk
1 banana
2 tablespoons marmalade
3 glasses of water between breakfast and mid-morning
      snack

Total: 470 calories, 3 grams fat, and 2½ milligrams cholesterol—
so if you want to have a swipe of cream cheese (low-fat) on your
muffin, go ahead—1½ fruit servings, 3 grain servings, 1 dairy
serving

Mid-morning snack target: 150 calories and less than 20 grams of fat

MENU

1 cup fresh green grapes
1 graham cracker (½ ounce)
8 ounces water

Total: 170 calories, 2 grams fat, 0 milligrams cholesterol; 2 fruit servings, less than ½ grain serving

Lunch target: maximum 550 calories and 12 grams of fat

MENU

1 pita pocket
½ serving veggie basics with yogurt dill dip (see page 190)
3 ounces tuna in water
1 smoothie (see page 186)
3 glasses of water between lunch and dinner

Total: 523 calories, 4 grams fat, 42 milligrams cholesterol; 1 grain serving, 3 vegetable servings, 2–3 fruit servings, 1 meat serving

Mid-afternoon snack target: 200 calories and minimal fat

MENU

1 strawberry frappe (see page 185)

Total: 97 calories, 1 gram fat; 2½ fruit servings

Dinner target: maximum 800 calories and 20 grams of fat

½ *roast skinless chicken*
1 *cup broccoli spears, steamed*
1 *cup noodles with 1 serving marinara sauce*
1 *tossed salad with balsamic dressing*
1 *serving fruit dessert (see page 189)*

Total: 725 calories, 13 grams fat, 140 milligrams cholesterol;
2 meat servings, 2–3 grain servings, 3–4 vegetable servings,
1–2 fruit servings

For the day you've had 23 grams of fat, 185 milligrams of cholesterol, and just under 2,000 calories. A fine spa day— low fat, high energy, with 7 servings of vegetables, 6½ of grain, 8 of fruit, and 3 of meat. For a regular diet, however, don't hesitate to add another 10 grams of fat a day in *unsaturated* fats.

The diet is high enough in calories to fuel a moderately active woman, but if you are exercising strenuously, it's not enough, even if your goal is weight loss. When you're regularly putting out an extra 700 calories a day with tough aerobic exercise, you need to replace those calories with low-fat fuel.

Goals

20–30% of calories from fat = 48–80 grams fat
250 milligrams cholesterol
5 servings fresh vegetables (2.5 cups cooked)
3 servings fruit (3 pieces)
8 servings of grains, rice, and legumes
2 servings dairy (2 cups milk or yogurt)
no more than 2 servings of meat, fish, or poultry (4–6 ounces a day)

For a 2,200–2,400-Calorie Day

If you work out strenuously for an hour or more three or four days a week, you shouldn't be eating less than 2,200 calories a day—and chances are you can eat quite a lot more without gaining weight. But if you stop exercising for a period of time, reduce your intake proportionally.

Breakfast target: maximum of 800 calories and 20 grams of fat

MENU

8 ounces orange juice

1 serving fruit salad (page 188)

1 large bowl oatmeal

1 cup skim milk

¼ cup raisins

1 tablespoon honey

2 slices wheat toast

1 tablespoon butter

3 glasses of water between breakfast and lunch

Total: 700 calories, 12 grams fat, 38 milligrams cholesterol;
4 fruit servings, 3 grain servings, 1 dairy serving

Lunch target: maximum of 800 calories and 20 grams of fat

MENU

1 smoothie (page 186)

3–6 ounces grilled chicken

1 large burrito-size flour tortilla

½ cup cooked rice

1 serving black beans (page 192)

1 serving steamed vegetables (page 189)

unlimited salsa

sliced onions

2 tablespoons low-fat sour cream or grated low-fat cheese

Total: 634 to 776 calories, 9–12 grams fat; 81–154 milligrams
cholesterol; 2–3 vegetable servings, 2 fruit servings,
1–2 meat servings, 2 grain and legume servings, ½ dairy serving

Dinner target: maximum of 800 calories and 20 grams of fat

MENU

antipasto made with:

1 serving Tuscan bean salad (page 192)

assorted vegetables, artichoke hearts, asparagus, grilled peppers, grilled zucchini, grilled mushrooms (you can do them in the broiler with balsamic vinegar as a basting sauce—great flavor, no fat)

2 breadsticks

1 glass red wine

1 cup cooked angel-hair pasta

2–3 tablespoons garlic basil sauce (page 195)

6-ounce filet of sole in a parchment pouch with marinara sauce (see pages 197 and 196 respectively)

1 serving fruit dessert (page 189)

Total: 985 calories, 9 grams fat, 101 milligrams cholesterol; 3 vegetable servings, 1 fruit serving, 3 grain servings. (For an active person, this diet provides 3–4 poultry and fish servings, 8 grain servings, 6 vegetable servings, 7 fruit servings, and 1½ dairy servings.)

Ten

•

Spa-at-Home Programs

Now it's time for the fun! You can pick out the spa program that you want to try first: the *One-Hour Personal Spa* for you alone; the *Half-Day Treatment Program* for one—with suggested variations if you want to enjoy it with a partner; the *Full-Day Program for Two* (or more); the *Weekend Getaway Special* designed to give you, and whomever you choose to bring along, a total vacation.

Before you start, make sure you take the time to determine your skin type (pages 6–7) so you can select the appropriate treatment recipes. And don't hesitate to experiment with all the treatments designed for you.

The One-Hour Personal Spa

The only way truly to enjoy a one-hour spa is to have the recipes made up ahead of time or to buy the products that you like and have them at hand. Then you can devote the most amount of time to enjoying the treatments.

Aerobic interlude—10-minute stretch and warm-up
   #1 Stretching (page 145), including the Big Body Bend, Side Stretch, Waist Stretch, Shoulder and Arm Rotation, Neck Noodle, Calf Flex, and Achilles' Tendon Warm-Up

Cleanse, compress face—3 minutes
   Select cleanser for your skin type (page 25–28) or use aloe vera gel applied gently with your fingers and wiped off with damp cotton balls. Then select compress recipe for your skin type (page 28–30).

Normal skin cleansers
oatmeal or yogurt honey cleanser

Normal skin compress choices
peppermint, fennel, or chamomile tea; ylang-ylang essential oil

Dry skin cleansers
cocoa butter or oatmeal milk

Dry skin compress choices
parsley or chamomile tea with honey; rose, carrot, or peppermint (not for pregnant women) essential oils

Oily skin cleansers
lemon-honey aloe or
tomato cucumber

Oily skin compress choices
sage, chamomile, or
lemon balm tea;
ylang-ylang, lavender,
and basil (not for preg-
nant women) essential
oils

*Blemished or sensitive skin
cleansers*
peppermint yogurt or
aloe vera with essential
oils

*Blemished or sensitive skin
compress choices*
chamomile, lemon balm
valerian, or lime flower
tea;
chamomile and floral
waters

Soak—10 minutes

Draw your bath before you cleanse and compress your face. Choose whichever one appeals to you.

Relaxing soak	*Moisturizing soaks*	*Aromatic soaks*
(page 79)	(page 81)	(page 74)
chamomile, basil,	milk and honey	cider vinegar
valerian, or	or oatmeal milk	
lavender		

Face and ear self-massage—5 minutes

Follow instructions for face and ear massage (page 117); use a moisturizing lotion suited to your skin type, or use a few drops of vitamin E oil, on your fingertips to smooth the massage. When done, cleanse face lightly with aloe vera gel and damp cotton balls. Rinse with luke-warm water and pat dry. Then . . .

Mask/Tone/Moisturize—15–25 minutes

Choose whichever one suits your skin type.

Masks for normal skin	*Toner for normal skin*	*Moisturizer for normal skin*
avocado, jello surprise, fruit, seaweed, or aromatherapy	witch hazel lemon-mint	lotion formulated for normal skin, or chamomile or ylang-ylang aromatherapy
Masks for oily skin	*Toner for oily skin*	*Moisturizer for oily skin*
eggwhite aloe, lemon banana, cucumber, or aromatherapy	witch hazel lemon-mint	not recommended
Masks for dry skin	*Toner for dry skin*	*Moisturizer for dry skin*
honey almond, mayonnaise, milk and cookies, or aromatherapy	diluted cider vinegar	humectants, or lotions with rose or carrot essential oils
Masks for blemished or sensitive skin	*Toner for blemished or sensitive skin*	*Moisturizer for blemished or sensitive skin*
beta-carotene, banana chamomile, tomato, or aromatherapy	aloe vera chamomile	oil-free and mildly antiseptic lotions or lotions with lavender, bergamot, rose, and carrot essential oils

Meditate—5 minutes

To end the program, follow the 5-minute guided meditation on page 130.

Spa Beverage—Once you're done, enjoy a refreshing and energizing Fruit Frappe (page 185)

or

Thigh Therapy—20 minutes (page 72–76)

Step One: Choose the herbal or seaweed wrap

Step Two: Follow with the circulation-enhancing scrub

Step Three: The skin-toning splash

Step Four: The deep moisturizing honey treatment

Foot Massage—10 minutes

Follow the reflexology or general foot massage instructions on page 122–125. This is a massage you can easily give yourself.

Facial—30 minutes

Follow the complete 30-minute facial routine options outlined on page 54.

Meditate—5 minutes

To end the program, follow the 5-minute guided meditation on page 130.

Spa Beverage—Once you're done, enjoy a refreshing and energizing Fruit Frappe (page 185).

The Half-Day Treatment Program

This is an outline for one person. If you're enjoying the spa with a friend, see the Half-Day with Partner on page 218. Begin this in the morning or at midday. It runs a little more than 3½ hours.

Aerobics—10 minutes
  #1 Stretching—Use this limbering-up routine to awaken your body and senses so you're more receptive to the spa treatments (see pages 145–47).

Breakfast or lunch—20 minutes
  Try the recipes and foods starting on page 183.

60-Minute Facial—Follow the 60-minute facial routine options outlined on page 55.

Body Wrap—20 minutes
  Choose whichever one appeals to you.

For moisturizing	*For energizing*	*Calming wrap*
(pages 89–91)	(pages 91–93)	(pages 93–94)
avocado oatmeal	rosemary oil	aromatherapy
mud wrap	wrap	
milk and honey	citrus spritz	
wrap		

Soak—15 minutes

Choose whichever one appeals to you.

Relaxing soaks	*Moisturizing soaks*	*Aromatic soaks*
(pages 79–81)	(pages 81–83)	(page 85)
chamomile, basil,	milk and honey	cider vinegar
valerian, or	or oatmeal milk	
lavender		

Snack—10 minutes

Make sure you drink at least 16 ounces of spring-water and then make yourself a Smoothie Plus or Vegetable Drink (pages 186 and 187).

Foot treatment and massage—30 minutes

Follow the instructions for foot treatments and the foot massage on pages 122–25

Meditation—15 minutes

Color Meditation (pages 132–35) or if you have time the 30- to 60-minute *Journey of the Peaceful Rest Meditation* (pages 135–38).

Half-Day with Partner

If two people are doing the half-day, you may want to change the routine so both receive a full-body massage. One possible timeline runs:

Walk or jog 2 miles—around 20 to 40 minutes, depending on your speed

If you can't go outside to exercise or don't have a treadmill, follow the exercise routine beginning on page 142—select 10 minutes of stretching exercises, 10 minutes of toning, 10 minutes of aerobics, and 10 minutes of after-workout stretching. Drink 16 ounces of springwater when done.

Breakfast or Lunch—20 minutes

30-Minute Facial—Both people do it at the same time. Follow the routine options on page 54.

Body Wrap—20–40 minutes

Depending on your facilities, you can do these one at a time or together. See pages 89 to 94 for recipes and instructions. Choose whichever one appeals to you.

For moisturizing	*For energizing*	*Calming wrap*
avocado oatmeal	*and stimulating*	aromatherapy
mud or milk and	rosemary oil	
honey wrap	wrap or citrus	
	spritz	

Soak—10 minutes

Choose whichever one appeals to you.

Relaxing soaks	*Moisturizing soaks*	*Aromatic soaks*
(pages 79–81)	(pages 81–83)	(page 85)
chamomile, basil,	milk and honey	cider vinegar
valerian, or	or oatmeal milk	
lavender		

Person #1 enjoys the tub while . . .

Meditation—15 minutes

Person #2 enjoys a *Color Meditation* (pages 132–35)

Full-Body Massage—40 minutes

Person #1 receives a massage (pages 107–26)

Snack—10 minutes

When the first massage is over, both people should drink 16 ounces of springwater and have a Fruit Frappe (pages 185–86).

Meditation—15 minutes

Person #1 does the *Color Meditation* while . . .

Soak—10 minutes

Person #2 takes a soak in the tub.

Full-Body Massage—40 minutes

Person #2 receives a massage.

Shower and Scrub—10 minutes

Both may want to end with a refreshing shower using the sugar scrub on page 95.

Full-Day Spa for Two

A day or two before you are scheduled to have a spa day for two, you may want to look at the Spa Cuisine chapter and determine what meal plan you two would like to follow for the day. Then do some advance shopping and preparation so you can cook and enjoy your meals without a hassle. But this routine doesn't have to be for two. If you want to do a full day of treatments for you alone—what a wonderful break from a hectic life—you can modify easily what follows.

Spa Breakfast—20 minutes
    Follow menu guidelines on pages 200-210.

Exercise Routine—40 minutes
    You may choose to walk or jog 2 miles—around 20–40 minutes, depending on your speed. If you can't go outside to exercise or don't want to, follow the exercise routine beginning on page 142—select 10 minutes of stretching exercises, 10 minutes of toning, 10 minutes of aerobics, and 10 minutes of after-workout stretching.

Water Break—Drink at least 16 ounces of springwater.

Soak—15 minutes
    Choose whichever one appeals to you.

Relaxing soaks	*Moisturizing soaks*	*Aromatic soaks*
(pages 79–81)	(pages 81–83)	(page 82)
chamomile, basil, valerian, or lavender	milk and honey or oatmeal milk	cider vinegar

Snack—10 minutes
> Enjoy a Smoothie Plus (page 186).

Facial—60 minutes
> Follow the facial routine options on page 55.

Lunch—30 minutes
> Try one of the recipes on pages 185–99. Drink at least 16 ounces of springwater.

Hair Repair, Hands, and Feet Treats—30 minutes

For hair repair (pages 57–65), select one:
> *Dry scalp and hair treatment*
> *Oily hair and scalp treatment*
> *Herbal hair treatments*
> *Shine enhancing treatments*

For hands (pages 65–67), select one:
> Deep moisturizing
> Nail therapy

For feet (pages 68–70), select one:
> *Relaxing soak*
> *Callus removal*
> *To cool hot tired feet*
> *To soften skin and smooth heels*

Thigh Therapy—20–30 minutes (pages 72–76)
> Step One: Choose the herbal or seaweed wrap
> Step Two: Follow with the circulation-enhancing scrub
> Step Three: The skin-toning splash
> Step Four: The deep moisturizing honey treatment

Water Break—Drink at least 16 ounces of springwater.

Full-Body Massage—90 minutes total—each person's lasts about 40 minutes (pages 107–26)

Water Break—Drink at least 16 ounces of springwater.

Shower Scrub—10 minutes
   For both of you when you are finished with the massages. Use the sugar scrub on page 95. Afterward, moisturize your body all over with aloe vera gel or a lotion formulated for your skin type. For dry skin apply lotion to still-damp skin to hold in moisture.

Meditation—15 minutes
   Color Meditation (pages 132–35)

For those of you who are having dinner as part of the spa day, try the Fish Fantastic recipe on page 197.

Weekend Getaway Special

A day or two before you are scheduled to have a spa weekend, you may want to look at the Spa Cuisine chapter and determine what meal plan you two would like to follow. Then do some advance shopping and preparation so you can cook and enjoy your meals without a hassle. The first day runs from 9 A.M. until around 4 P.M. You can, of course, alter it to fit your schedule. The second day is a bit shorter. Also, this doesn't have to be for two. If you want to do the treatments for you alone—what a wonderful break from a hectic life—you can modify easily what follows.

Day One
9 A.M. Exercise—60 minutes
  You may choose to walk or jog for 45 minutes—if so begin with *#1 Stretching* routine on pages 145-47 and finish with the *#4 Advanced Stretching* on pages 155–58. If you can't go outside to exercise or don't want to, follow the exercise routine beginning on page 142—do 15 minutes of stretching exercises, 15 of toning, 15 of aerobics, and 15 of after-workout stretching on pages 155–58. Drink 16 ounces of springwater when done.

Breakfast—30 minutes
  Drink at least 16 ounces of springwater.

Soak—15 minutes

Choose whichever one appeals to you.

Relaxing soaks	*Moisturizing soaks*	*Aromatic soaks*
(pages 79–81)	(pages 81–83)	(page 85)
chamomile, basil,	milk and honey	cider vinegar
valerian, or	or oatmeal milk	
lavender		

Body Wrap—20–40 minutes

Depending on your facilities, you can do these one at a time or together. See pages 87–94 for recipes and instructions. Choose whichever one appeals to you.

For moisturizing	*For energizing*	*Calming wrap*
avocado oatmeal	*and stimulating*	aromatherapy
mud or milk and	rosemary oil	
honey wrap	wrap or citrus	
	spritz	

Water Break—Drink at least 16 ounces of springwater.

Feet, Hand, and Elbow Treatments—30 minutes (optional now, if you have enough time before you would like to have lunch)

Hand treatments	*Foot treatments*
(pages 65–67)	(pages 68–70)
Deep moisturizing	Relaxing soak
Nail repair	Remove calluses
	Cool hot, tired feet
	Soften skin and smooth heels

3-in-1 Elbow therapy (pages 71–72)
Step One: Softening compress
Step Two: Remove dry, dead skin
Step Three: Moisturize

Lunch—30–60 minutes
    Enjoy sampling the spa recipes beginning on page 183. Drink at least 16 ounces of springwater.

Facial—60 minutes
    Follow the facial routine options on pages 51–55.

Stretching Exercises—10 minutes
    #1 Stretching routine (pages 145–47).

Full Body Massage—90 minutes for both people (pages 107–26).

Water Break—Drink at least 16 ounces of springwater.

Feet, Hand, and Elbow Treatments—30 minutes (optional now, if you didn't do them before lunch).

Meditation—30–60 minutes
    Journey of the Peaceful Rest (pages 135–38).

Spa Dinner—when hungry

Day Two
9 A.M. *Walking Meditation (page 138)—*
40 minutes

If you can't or don't want to go outside, you can replace it with either an extended *Color Meditation* (pages 132–35) or the *Journey of the Peaceful Rest* (pages 135–38).

Breakfast—30 minutes

Cleanse, Compress, Tone, and Moisturize Your Complexion—15 minutes

For normal skin

Cleanser: yogurt and honey (page 26) Compress: chamomile tea (page 29)	Toner: witch hazel lemon-mint (page 44)	Moisturizer: lotion formulated for normal skin, or with chamomile or ylang-ylang essential oils

For oily skin

Cleanser: lemon, honey, aloe vera wash (page 27) Compress: chamomile tea (page 29)	Toner: witch hazel lemon-mint (page 44)	Moisturizer: not recommended

For dry skin

Cleanser: oatmeal milk (page 27)
Compress: chamomile honey tea (page 29)

Toner: not recommended

Moisturizer: humectants or lotions with rose or carrot essential oils

For blemished or sensitive skin

Cleanser: peppermint yogurt (page 28)
Compress: chamomile tea or eucalyptus and lavender essential oils (page 30)

Toner: aloe vera chamomile (page 45)

Moisturizer: oil-free and mildly antiseptic lotions or lotions with lavender, bergamot, rose, and carrot essential oils

Hair Treatment—30 minutes

Select one or more treatments (pages 57–65) that work with your hair type.

Dry hair and scalp treatment
Oily hair and scalp treatment
Herbal hair treatments
Shine enhancing treatments

Shower Scrub—10 minutes

Use the exfoliating treatments in the facial chapter for an all-over scrub. Choose the one that suits your skin type.

Normal skin	Dry skin	Oily skin
(page 32)	(page 33)	(page 34)
oatbran egg yolk,	oatmeal yogurt,	aloe vera oatmeal,
almond honey	sugar scrubs	banana cornmeal
cream		

Honey Body-Moisturizing Treatment—10 minutes

After you're done with the shower scrub, turn off the shower but remain in the shower stall.

Pat your skin dry and then spread it with honey (using a plastic squeeze jar). Spread honey all over with your hands and allow to sit for 10 minutes.

If you get chilled, wrap your body in a plastic wrapper such as you use for a body wrap, or a terry-cloth robe—the honey will wash out. It's important not to become chilled or your muscles will tense up.

Reflexology Foot Massage—10 minutes

Using the reflexology chart on pages 124–25, massage the areas that correspond to any achy or stiff areas of your body, such as lower back, back of the leg, neck, or shoulders.

Lunch—30–60 minutes

Enjoy sampling the spa recipes on pages 185–99. Drink at least 16 ounces of springwater.

Hand Treatment—20 minutes

Use the *deep moisturizing* treatment on pages 66–67 if you need more time to digest your lunch before you and your partner can give each other a face massage. That will take about half an hour (pages 117–19).

Exercise Routine—60 minutes

You may choose to walk or jog for 45 minutes—if so, begin with *#1 Stretching* routine on pages 145–47 and finish with *#4 Advanced Stretching* on pages 155–58. If you can't go outside to exercise or don't want to, follow the exercise routine beginning on page 142—do 15 minutes of stretching exercises, 15 of toning, 15 of aerobics, and 15 of after-workout stretching on pages 155–58.

Drink 16 ounces of springwater when done.

Soak—15 minutes

Choose whichever one appeals to you.

Relaxing soaks (pages 79–81) chamomile, basil, valerian, or lavender	*Moisturizing soaks* (pages 81–83) milk and honey or oatmeal milk	*Aromatic soaks* (page 85) cider vinegar

Snack—10 minutes

Enjoy a smoothie (page 186), a bowl of berries and low-fat yogurt, or some baked chips and salsa. Drink at least 16 ounces of springwater.

Full-Body Massage—90 minutes for each person to have a complete massage (pages 107–26).

Moisturizing Shower—10 minutes

After giving or receiving a massage, it feels great to have a relaxing, moisturizing shower. Try the sugar scrub on page 95.

Spa Dinner—whenever you get hungry

Resources and
Sources

◆

If you are looking for spa supplies and equipment, we suggest you contact the following sources:

You can reach The Wellness Center at 591 Albany Post Road, Hyde Park, NY 12538, or by calling 914-229-5560.

Massage and Spa Products
and Equipment

The Healing Touch video offers the basics of giving an effective whole-body massage: easy to follow, step-by-step instructions for massaging back, back of legs, neck, head and face, arms and hands, front of legs and feet, and abdomen. By Dale Grust, director of The Wellness Center. Cost: $29.95 plus $3 shipping. New York State residents add 8.25% sales tax; make checks payable to The Wellness Center.

The Wellness Center's own line of massage oils, and other products, such as aromatic candles, soaps, and loofah mitts, is available through mail order. For a catalog and order form please contact The Wellness Center at the address or phone number on page 230.

Customized at-home spa baskets are available through Maureen DiCorcia, director of spa services at The Wellness Center. Please test your skin type (see pages 6–7) before ordering so you can receive appropriate skin products.

The basic gift basket contains cleansing cream, exfoliant, mask, toner, moisturizer, and terry-cloth headband. $60 plus $5 shipping. (New York State residents please add 8.25% sales tax.)

Individual customized products, including salts, mineral mud body treatments, seaweed body treatments, herbal bath treatments, aromatherapy essential bath oils, and more, available upon request. Prices from $5.

To request an order form or to place an order, send check to Maureen DiCorcia, Director Spa Therapy, at the above address.

Aromatic Embrace NecCradle, an unscented pillow with rice and red cedar chips or scented with rice, rose petals, red cedar chips, oak moss, vetiver, German chamomile flowers, lavender flowers, marjoram, and lemongrass, can be heated in the microwave or conventional oven and used to relax or ease muscle pain all over the body. Great when used before a massage. Also works as cold pack. Available through The Wellness Center or by calling 800-943-8806. Cost: $29.95 (New York State residents add 8.25% sales tax) plus $4 shipping.

Great for self- or partnered massage, the **Thumper mini-pro,** a hand-held massager, costs around $240.00. It is the ultimate solution to chronically knotted or sore muscles. To order, contact The Wellness Center at the address or phone number on page 230, or call the manufacturer 800-848-6737.

For additional spa products you may want to write for the **Best of Nature** catalog. This supplier of professional products to massage therapists stocks everything from massage tools—electric and manual—to essential oils and heat packs. Call 800-228-6457 for a catalog or write to PO Box 3164, Long Branch, New Jersey 07740.

Meditation Tapes

Guided meditations are available on cassettes. The tape, with spoken word and music, includes a 20-minute guided relaxation and meeting with the higher self and a 20-minute chakra balancing and prosperity meditation. Cost: $11.95 (plus 8.25% sales tax for New York State residents). Make checks payable to Margaret Doner and send orders to The Wellness Center, 591 Albany Post Road, Hyde Park, NY 12538.

Herbal Information

American Botanical Council, PO Box 201660, Austin, Texas 78720-1660, is a nonprofit research and education center that offers a quarterly magazine, herbal education catalog, and other materials. To order products call: 800-373-7105. On the web: http://www.Herbalgram.org